GW00469585

From Cancer to Clear

my eight eye openers to improve your health

Julie Harrison

Copyright © 2015 Julie Harrison

All rights reserved.

ISBN-13: 978-0-9934916-0-3

Published by
Get Seriously Healthy

This book is the story of my personal journey from being diagnosed with breast cancer to achieving the best health and fitness in my life. It is offered for educational purposes only. Please note that I have no formal medical qualifications, and nothing in this book should be taken as medical advice. It is the reader's responsibility to seek appropriate medical advice from a qualified health professional of their choice before embarking on any of the suggestions.

No part or the whole of this book may be reproduced, distributed, transmitted or utilized (other than for reading by the intended reader) in ANY form (now known or hereafter invented) without prior written permission by the author, except by a reviewer, who may quote brief passages in a review. The unauthorized reproduction or distribution of this copyrighted work is illegal and punishable by law.

This book is dedicated to

Phillip Day

A man who has the courage of his convictions and who isn't afraid to tell the truth. Without him and his passion for genuinely helping people I am not sure if I would be on the path that I am travelling.

I would also like to thank...

John Shepherd for supporting my "wild and wacky" ideas.

My parents, Ann and John Booth, for always being there for me.

Steve Szubert for all his advice and support.

And all my wonderful kind and caring friends—you know who you are!

CONTENTS

Foreword

Too many of us are getting cancer now. The latest scary statistics state that one out of two people will hear those dreaded words.

I have been at the receiving end and I don't want that to happen to you. I was told I had breast cancer back in 2009 and this book shares my story to full recovery and better health than ever before, but more importantly how you can change your diet and lifestyle to avoid it happening to you. I did it the hard way but I will show you a much easier path, one that I wish I had had all those years ago.

Numerous people have followed my path and have found that life gets much easier and your health improves quickly if you follow a few simple steps, which is why I wrote this book.

Let me help you. Read on and see how they helped me and discover what has the most effect on your health.

Introduction: Lightning Strikes

*(the beginning of
my personal story)*

*Whatever your own story may be,
the foundations of health
are universal.
This book can help you.*

"You have cancer"

Those three devastating words became the catalyst for me to create my perfect life.

Although, it took me a while to see that. Even the initial shock crept in slowly.

It began in the spring of 2009. Investigating an itch near my armpit, I found a minuscule lump. Or so I thought. Despite more prodding around I couldn't find it again. I forgot about it until July 2009.

Another itch. This time the lump was quite easy to find. It was still smaller than the size of a pea. More like the size of a grape seed. So I hesitated to trouble my doctor with it. But I decided to go for convenience since I was on holiday from work and would not need to take time off. That was me all over; not wanting to inconvenience anyone.

That same afternoon my doctor assured me that it did not feel like a cancerous lump, but she wanted me to have it checked further, just to be on the safe side.

Within a week I was at the hospital. Nothing was picked up on the mammogram but there was a murmur on the ultrasound. Both the examining doctor and ultrasound technician thought a biopsy should be done—to be on the safe side—even though everything looked normal and there was "no need to worry."

But how could I not worry? The only way I could really feel "on the safe side" would be if they could clearly rule out any need for further checks.

Ten fretful days later I returned for the biopsy result. There was abnormal cell activity.

They wanted a further core biopsy to determine if it was cancerous. This time there was no reassurance of being "on the safe side".

Ten more days seemed like forever.

I knew it was cancer when I was finally being ushered into the doctor's office. There was a nurse and another doctor there too. None of them looked like they were there for a party. For a month now reassurances of being "on the safe side" had been wearing thin.

To hear those three fateful words, "**You have cancer**," was no surprise. But expectation did not diminish how it felt.

Totally desolate.

My mission

From that place of knowing what it feels like to be the target of those words—"you have cancer"—I have made it my mission to help others who have landed in that same hell. And hopefully even help you stay out of there altogether.

I learnt to climb out of it the complicated way, figuring things out as I stumbled along, making many mistakes along the way. Looking back I can now trace a path that would have made things much simpler for me.

I want to show you this more simple path. A way that can bring you the most benefit from the least effort—I believe in value for money.

We tend to overlook "simple" and brush it aside. That's how things become complicated and difficult.

I want to help you steer around "complicated" and take you deeper into "simple".

I want to show you an easy way to make health a normal part of your daily life.

Not just cancer

Along my journey, I became more sharply aware of and interested in the health challenges faced by others. I wanted to know what they were doing that was working to get them healthy again. I came to realise that cancer is not the only disease that can wreak such sheer devastation on a life.

More importantly, I came to learn that whatever the name doctors put on the condition, the very same principles can offer the key to recovery and restored health.

It's not that surprising really when you consider that it's the same body whatever the illness. So why would a holistic approach—one that takes into account the workings of the whole body—not be beneficial?

I had already found clear evidence of this in myself.

Years earlier I had been in a skydiving accident that, by all accounts, should have finished me off or at least permanently debilitated me. That's a story for another day. The thing is, I did recover from that accident, but only up to a point. I was left with constant pain that I had to live with every day.

Until that is I started implementing some of the holistic approaches intended to help me overcome cancer. One day, I noticed that my pain had vanished. It has never returned.

So, based on my own experience and the experience of others that I see repeated again and again, I cannot help but firmly believe that my Eight Eye Openers I'm going to share with you can be helpful whatever the health challenge you might be facing.

Of course, I do have to say that I am not medically qualified and I am not giving medical advice here—I am simply sharing information—and you should always consult a suitably qualified medical practitioner of your choice, on how to apply any information in your own specific case.

Even if you consider yourself "healthy", you could be amazed at the improvement that can come from putting these principles into practice right now.

Why wait for a disease to take hold? Why not keep a step ahead and improve your health right now?

Where I am now

For me, this journey has turned out to be the most positive and rewarding experience. Along the way, I have met amazing people who have taught me how to truly take control of my life. Looking back I can now see that "Before Cancer" (BC), I had only been going through the motions of being in control.

As my journey continues, I have never felt as fit, healthy and happy. I love life and I love learning to live it more joyfully.

The passion that drives me forward is a hunger for the feeling of looking back and seeing I have helped you create in your life the same transformation that I enjoy in mine. I have learnt so much, and now I want to pass this knowledge onto you.

I will show you how you can make simple changes that can raise your life to a whole new level of health and joy— whether you have cancer or not.

The probability is that you have a 50% chance of being at the receiving end of those 3 words at some point in your life. I want to help you stay on the right side of that statistic.

This is the book I so wish I'd had from the start.

But enough about my story, for now. The primary aim of this book is to help you change the story of your own life for the better. Let's begin that now. Enjoy your journey—to your best of health.

My Eight Eye Openers

JULIE HARRISON

Eye Opener 1: Ask Questions

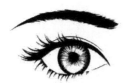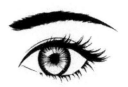

*Good decisions
depend on you having
the information
that's right for you
in your situation.*

Who do you trust?

We tend to turn to conventional sources for answers to vital questions about our health. But is it safe to blindly trust the answers we usually get from government, medical establishments and the media?

- Government—a game of politics played to win votes.
- Medicine—a game dominated by drugs companies playing to win big bucks.
- Media—a game of sound bites and fear stirring headlines played to win ratings.

All games in which we are pawns.

I used to be one of the many who blindly trusts. Until I was told I had breast cancer.

I have never felt so powerless as I did at that moment when it dawned on me that my very life was now in the hands of other people.

When those fated words—"you have cancer"—are directed at you, a riot of emotions runs through your body. Each fighting for a top place. I think the winner for me, was a screaming panic of, "Get it out! Get it out quick!"

Your first step

If you have been or ever are told you have cancer, there's something you really need to know.

***You can take back control and feel powerful again.
You can start taking responsibility for your own life.***

As I came to learn, this is the first step.

Too many people will try to tell you what to do. Especially qualified medical people. Yet, rarely does their advice feel like it comes from the heart.

Often, they don't even look at you. They seem lost somewhere in their heads as if reading the script from some textbook they are supposed to follow.

Somewhere in that script is the Standard of Care prescribed by the UK National Health Service. But somehow, a feeling of being cared for fails to come across. I often felt like just another number in the statistics.

Until I learned to take responsibility for myself and to start asking questions of others.

Was this meant to happen to me?

This enigmatic question still puzzles me to this day.

At the moment the diagnosis was announced to me I was instantly possessed by a feeling of choking panic. Yet, deep at the centre of that feeling, I was also aware of an other-worldly sense of peace.

It was as though I had always known I would get cancer.

In the years since then, I have gained a conviction that this life is no accident. I know that I signed up for my life and all that I experience in it.

Could it be that getting cancer was part of the plan?

But right at that moment, I had questions to ask of the consultant, who had effectively just told me that I was going to die—and most probably much sooner than I had ever thought I might.

Inner Wisdom

At moments like that, when time itself suddenly becomes painfully scarce, we can easily fall from acting out of a place of clarity to reacting from a place of fear.

With hindsight, I can now see that at those times when I acted from a place of fear, I failed to listen to my inner wisdom, no matter how loudly it cried out to me. At one such time, I agreed to a surgery which cost me my ovaries—more about that, later.

At those times when I have listened, my inner wisdom has always proven itself to me. I now have no shadow of a doubt that it pays to be still and to listen and to follow my inner wisdom. Later I will share with you some of the tools I learned to use, that will help you listen to your own inner wisdom.

Not that it was easy. Refusing radiotherapy was the hardest

decision of my life: a tough battle that raged inside and out, between my own fears and those of the medical profession and my family and my friends.

Family and friends

Just telling family members that I had breast cancer was a tough task to face up to. Dealing with their emotions and fears, even more so. But at least it helped deflect the focus from my own fears.

And I was no longer alone.

My wonderful brother Mark, when I broke the news to him he immediately did what guys do. Women talk and share and find deep value in just the emotional connection. We are not necessarily seeking to fix something. But for men, sharing a problem is taken as an invitation to figure out a practical solution.

So Mark's immediate response was to get a friend of his to call me. A friend who ran a counselling group for women with breast cancer.

The strangest advice from a stranger

Within five minutes a total stranger was offering me her time and energy—a part of her life—to help me save mine.

Judy was simply being there for me, listening. She gave me all her contact details and made it clear that I was not to hesitate if I ever needed to contact her.

She had advice available too, though only if I wanted it. But before ending that first conversation, Judy did advise me:

"Stop eating dairy."

Stop eating dairy? At that time, those words conflicted totally with what I had been brought up to believe.

How about you? "Stop eating dairy." How does that make you feel?

We *need* dairy! Without the calcium, our bones will crumble! Dairy is *essential* to a balanced diet!

Or is it? Find out more in Eye Opener Eight.

Eureka!

This was my turning point.

I started to ask questions.

Google has become one of my most beloved friends. Without the internet, it might have taken fifty years to achieve what I did, in barely five. Without the internet to help me find answers to my questions, I would most likely not be here now.

You have your life in your hands

I am in awe of Professor Jane Plant, who managed to clear herself of cancer before the days of the internet. Jane's breast cancer returned 5 times and despite 35 radiotherapy treatments, irradiation to induce the menopause and chemotherapy treatments she was told she had only months left to live. Her fabulous book *Your Life in Your Hands* goes into detail about her main discovery and that was how and why dairy should be avoided. Jane stopped eating her 2 yoghurts a day and all other dairy and within 6 weeks the solid lump, the size of half a small boiled egg sticking out of her neck had gone.

Later, I will share with you how I learned to use the internet effectively. In particular, I want to show you how not to get fooled by the fake information websites that are out there (often funded by the big pharmaceutical companies).

It all began when I spent a couple of hours exploring the issue of eating dairy. I began my search with an open mind. By the end of it, my mind was firmly set—I never wanted to consume dairy ever again.

Bigger questions

Next, I started to question my beliefs about cancer and its treatments. This was still a totally terrifying topic for me. At that point, I still desperately wanted the surgery. I wanted that lump *out* of my body—NOW.

But my journey down the rabbit hole had started. Once down there, you find it's a labyrinth. I was led around in circles—often the same ones more than once. I hit dead ends.

As well as spending hours at a time online, I'm sure I became one of Amazons top customers and lost count of the books I devoured. My best friend even gave me a massive bookcase to house them all.

The quality of the information I found ranged from awesome to abysmal. Here in this book, my aim is to share with you the best and the essential from what I have discovered through years of research and used successfully. I feel your urgency. I want to save you time.

But still, it is never easy. Please be gentle on yourself. Start slowly and take on board just the changes you feel you can cope with. Take things step by step.

Also, learn to ask for what you really want. When you are feeling vulnerable, it's hard to tell people how you feel. But the more you can do that, the more others can be there for you.

The greatest kindness

John, my boyfriend, has been an absolute marvel. Throughout the long wait for the results of my medical tests, he patiently listened with an open heart as I shared the discoveries from my research.

The day I was first diagnosed coincided with one of the days he had his children staying with him. I would never dream of asking him to cancel that.

I remember sitting alone in my lounge feeling overwhelmed by what was going to happen to me. I cried and cried feeling totally alone. Just thinking about it was exhausting. I fell asleep with the tears still rolling down my cheeks.

Amidst my strange dreams, I became aware of a pair of hands gently resting on my knees. I opened my eyes to see the man I loved kneeling in front of me, his eyes warm and soft with such a caring look flowing from them.

He had arranged for a babysitter to stay over with his children so that he could be with me.

I will remember that kindness for the rest of my life.

My first big mistake

When we talked about the operation itself, I told John

that "Yes" I would like him to come with me to the hospital, but urged him to go back to work as soon as I was settled in. Not wanting to put him out.

That was such a mistake.

Waiting to be called in for the operation.... Waiting...... Waiting......

Never in my whole life had I felt so desolately lonely and afraid; it was worse than being told you have cancer.

Waiting..... Four hours of trying to keep my mind from thoughts of how disfigured I would be after the operation. Or if I would even survive.

Don't be brave. Ask for what you need. I needed John.

After my first op

The surgeon told me afterwards, he'd had to cut out a lump the size of an egg from my breast. But I was fortunate. The lump had been to the side of the breast, so removing it had little effect on the appearance. Apart from the scars, it would be hardly noticeable.

What amazed me was that before surgery my bra cup size was A or AA. Logically, losing so much tissue should have had a profound effect—yet still, both breasts looked the same size.

That remains one of the mysteries of the Universe, and a good reason to say. "Thank you, Universe"

What next?

By now, I was getting comfortable with the dairy-free diet I had proudly adopted. I asked a nurse at the hospital for more information about what foods she'd recommend I eat.

She told me that nothing would make any difference and that cutting out dairy was a bad idea, a really bad idea.

That strengthened my resolve to start questioning whatever I was told by the medical profession.

I asked questions that were awkward for them to answer. Remember at the end of the day, we are the ones who have to live with the results of any decisions. So my advice is to ask away, regardless.

Six weeks (and lots more research) later, I had an

appointment with the oncologist to discuss chemotherapy, radiotherapy and drugs. I had lots of questions, but he quickly made me feel very foolish for even suggesting taking any natural treatments.

I remember asking him about Indol 3 Carbinol, a natural supplement which, from my research, seemed to offer the same or better protection against the cancer returning than the Tamoxifen he was offering.

He had never heard of it and wasn't interested in even discussing anything other than the cut, burn and poison strategy that he had been trained in.

So I turned my questions to the long-term effects of radiotherapy.

I was told that records were not kept.

I was outraged that "experts" expected me to accept without question such a drastic treatment, when they were ignorant of the long-term effects—and seemingly not even interested in knowing.

A better-informed view

At that time, I went to hear a talk by Phillip Day, an investigative journalist who travels the world to share the truths he has discovered about cancer and its treatments. During the interval, I approached him, quickly explained my case and asked if he thought I should have the radiotherapy that my oncologist insisted was essential.

He looked me in the eye and said: "Absolutely not".

Based on his talk, I very much respected Phillip Day and his opinions. So I continued to search for more information on what radiotherapy actually does to the body.

At the same time, the oncologist had made it very clear that to be effective, the radiotherapy had to be done soon, so I went back to the hospital to be measured up for it. Although I still wasn't sure that radiotherapy was the right thing. My research was not yet finished.

My tears flooded out while I was waiting to be measured up for the treatment. Every part of my body felt like it was screaming at me to get out of that hospital, that I shouldn't be having this done to me.

But everyone was telling me that I must. It was hard, going against all that I had been taught to believe in. It was harder going against my body crying out to live and to live well.

The actual measuring procedure was totally painless and the staff were lovely, although they didn't like me questioning them at all.

The process was completed by my being tattooed with two tiny black dots, to make it easier for the radiographer to set up the machine each time I was supposed to go back for radiotherapy.

I was told the tattoos would be permanent, but thankfully that was another thing they got wrong. The dots have faded now. It's as if my body is telling me that they are not needed.

Decision

As soon as I was home I had made my decision. I was *not* going to submit myself to radiotherapy. I was, at last, starting to trust my instinctive inner wisdom.

A very good decision.

My second big mistake

However, because the cancer I had was oestrogen receptive I was strongly advised to have my ovaries removed.

I went ahead with that.

A very bad decision.

After waking up from that operation, I carried on with the book I'd been reading: "Knockout" by Suzanne Somers.

Only fifteen minutes further into that book, I learned just how important a woman's ovaries are to her.

I don't usually do "if only", but if I had just read that part of the book *before* the operation.

I would have cancelled it and carried on with more research. However, I believe everything happens for a reason and regrets aren't that helpful.

Ask questions—don't be afraid of hurting somebody's feelings. It is your body and you need to have the facts and be comfortable with the decisions you are making.

KEY ACTION POINTS

- Take responsibility for your own life. At the end of the day, it *is* your life.
- Question everything—you have a right to know.
- Remember that "experts" are expert only in their own field.
- Learn to listen to your own inner wisdom—your gut feeling. It's usually the very first thought or feeling you have before the mind tries to rationalise it.
- Keep an open mind. Suspend judgement and be willing to find out more.
- Ask for help; especially from people who have been through the same as you.
- Tell people how you feel, also tell people what you need from them. How else can they know?
- Forgive yourself your mistakes—keep learning from them and move forward.

JULIE HARRISON

Eye Opener 2: Are You Drinking Real Water?

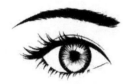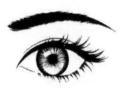

*After learning to ask questions,
the next step is to not
take simple things for granted—
like water.
Here's the "acid" test.*

Update (2018) to Eye Opener 2

The following chapter is how my journey progressed. However, now I don't drink alkaline water and wouldn't recommend this method. For simplicity, I'd recommend a whole house water filter. That way you are drinking, bathing and washing your clothes in pure water.

I'm not frightened to change my mind when I find out new information.

What makes disease possible?

Once you start to apply the holistic view to investigating the root causes of ill health, you very soon notice the same culprit popping up everywhere.

Too much acidity.

Most diseases can only take hold in a body that is too acidic. Since Western diets tend to be highly acidic, is it any wonder we are suffering more and more ill health?

We might be living longer, but it's rare to find anyone over the age of 60 (or even 50) not on some form of medication. It seems to be a way of life that has become accepted as inevitable. It doesn't have to be.

We will come back to diet in Eye Opener 8. The problem begins with something much more basic, so much so that we tend to overlook it.

Water.

We drink it, cook with it, wash in it and use it to clean our clothes, our homes, our cars... We rely on water for everything. When it flows at the turn of a tap we take it for granted.

But your health is at serious risk unless you take steps to ensure that your body is awash with water—both inside and out. Not just any water, but healthy, living water.

Most likely it isn't. Therefore, that leaves you wide open to the onset of disease.

You *are* dehydrated

I know. I too, dismissed that as a silly notion when I first heard it. How can I be dehydrated? I don't even feel thirsty.

But feeling parched only comes at a seriously advanced stage of dehydration.

- Do you tire easily, get dizzy or have frequent headaches?
- Do you suffer skin problems, especially dryness and inexplicable itches?
- Do you get constipated?
- Is your urine dark yellow or amber, rather than a light golden colour or clear?
- Do you find it difficult to turn on the tears when you feel like crying?

All of those could be signs of dehydration. As always, check with your doctor if any symptoms persist.

Some facts about snacks

Coming back to the point of rarely feeling thirsty, do you frequently find yourself feeling peckish between meals? Often, that feeling is actually thirst which we mistake for hunger.

Try this experiment. Next time you feel like snacking because you are "hungry", have just a glass of water. And wait.

You'll most likely find you have lost your feeling of "hunger" because you have given your body what it was really asking for—water.

Quite likely, you will still have a snack as well, from force of habit. Keep repeating this experiment and watch your food cravings diminish as your body starts to feel more satisfied with the amount of water you are giving it.

The bigger problem with snacks is that we tend to have them with a beverage of some kind—tea, coffee, coke, alcohol... None of those fluids counts as water. Rather, your body identifies them as "polluted" water and sets about trying to get rid of it. A process which uses water—which is why too much of any beverage actually *de*-hydrates your body.

So, an important basic step towards better health is to grow the habit of drinking more water and more often. Regardless of how unnecessary you might feel that is right now, try it and see the difference: more energy, less dizziness, fewer headaches... Remember that list of signs of dehydration?

But hydration is not just about getting water into your stomach. It goes way beyond that.

Why you get tired too easily

Most of us are dehydrated at the cellular level. Without diving into the fascinating science of what goes on down there, trust me that no cell can function in a healthy way without plenty of water.

So what does your body do when it is short of water? To survive, it has to ration what is available. That ensures the more important cells—in places like the heart and brain—get the water they need. It also means that less important cells have to go without.

In any state other than full hydration, your body has no choice but to shut down a percentage of the cells in less vital places like your limbs. It does that by coating those cells with cholesterol. Those cells are revisited from time to time and given a tiny squirt of water—but only just enough to keep them barely alive. Those cells remain shut off and unavailable for healthy functioning.

That's why you feel aches and pains all over and get tired long before you should—all because your body is dehydrated at the cellular level.

Drinking more is not enough

Just drinking more water is not enough because you can't drink it straight into your cells. It has to be taken in through your gut.

Which is a good thing.

Your gut is your first line of defence in your immune system. Before it lets anything into your body, your gut needs to be sure that what you are giving it is the real deal. And that applies to water too.

I have already mentioned how beverages, even though they are mostly water, can trigger your body to use water to get rid of them. For best health and full hydration, you need to make clean, living water your main beverage.

I would suggest, as a bare minimum that you filter all the water you use for drinking. That includes the water you use to make hot drinks, together with the water you cook with.

Just be sure to change the filter regularly.

Keeping things really clean

Skin is waterproof, right? That's why we don't dissolve in the rain, isn't it? So it doesn't matter what kind of water we wash in?

I'm afraid it does. Very much so.

Not only does your skin absorb into your body some of the water you wash in—along with what's in it—but it does so more readily, the warmer the water is. Because heat opens up your pores.

Any doubts you might have about this should quickly fade when you realise that nicotine patches and hormone therapy patches work for that very reason—because your skin *is* absorbent.

What's worrying here is that what comes into your body through the skin bypasses something vital I mentioned earlier—that first line of defence of your immune system that you have—your gut.

So, if the water you drink needs to be filtered before you take it into your body, what about the water you drench your skin with, some of which also gets absorbed? It may be only a little, but it goes straight into your body, along with whatever is in it.

The cheapest way to start filtering the water you wash in is a simple attachment for your shower head. Again, be sure to change the filter regularly.

You can go as far as installing systems that will filter every drop of water that runs through your house—an ideal scenario. But take care. You can go too far with filtering water and filter the "life" out of it.

For example, a reverse osmosis system filters out absolutely everything and leaves you with "dead" liquid. You then need to do something to add back the beneficial minerals that make water "alive".

What is "living" water?

Viktor Schauberger was a man of noble birth, growing up in Austria in the mid eighteen hundreds. Despite nobility, his family were poor and Viktor had to work hard to earn a living from the surrounding forests...

Don't worry; I haven't suddenly switched to writing a romantic novel!

The point is that this man was close to nature, which he studied with a passion. A particular passion of his was water—particularly its structure and the energy it contains.

Yes, water is actually an energy system. Viktor was also gifted with engineering skills and designed alternative energy devices based on implosion—vastly more environmentally friendly than destructive energy sources that use explosion.

Reading about Viktor Schauberger's life in a book called "Living Water" totally changed how I view the thing called water that we so take for granted.

One fact, in particular, is relevant here. As water passes through the network of pipes from the reservoirs to our homes, it loses its living energy.

What comes out of our taps is in fact dead. Very different from the living water we would draw from a natural well or spring. Natural water is alive with traces of essential minerals and organic compounds.

The wonders of water are further demonstrated through the famous work of Dr Emoto. If you haven't seen his photographs of water crystals and the beautiful shapes that living water makes compared to the distorted forms of dead water please search for the images on Google.

I heartily recommend that you make time to read more about the work of Viktor Schauberger and Dr Emoto. But right now, we have one pressing question above all else.

Can "dead" water come back to life?

Most of us have little choice but to use the dead liquid that comes out of our taps. We know we can filter out much of what was not put in by nature, but can we do anything to revive the living qualities of water that nature did intend for us?

Yes, we can.

You can re-energise your water by putting it through a vortex. But that comes after...

My secret weapon

At this point in our story of water, I bring in what I call my secret weapon and we also return to the big problem I mentioned at the start of this chapter: that most diseases can only take hold in a body that is too acidic.

You can do something about that. Simply by drinking water that has been alkalised.

Acidity and its opposite alkalinity are measured on the

pH scale. Extremes at either end of the scale will burn—such as battery acid with a low pH of around 1 and bleach with a high pH of around 14.

Now, body pH varies in different parts of the body, and also depends on what's going on in the body. For example, the stomach is very acidic during digestion, but that acidity has to be neutralised immediately the stomach passes its contents further down the line.

The important number here is the pH of your blood, the ideal range being between 7.36 and 7.44 (just a shade towards the alkaline side of a neutral 7). For the water you drink, the best pH is as close as possible to the ideal pH range of your blood.

The secret weapon I use for this is a water ionizer. You know how refreshing it is to be by the sea, or by a waterfall? That's the effect of the ions that abound around water in its natural, living, moving state.

An ioniser can revive that quality in plain tap water and the process also restores the water to an ideal pH.

The ionising unit fits easily via a tube onto your water taps and is very user-friendly. The one I use also filters the water. And to that, I have added a vortex funnel to re-energise it. That literally spins the water round to liven it up and get some air bubbles into it.

At a pinch, you can get some of the effects simply by flipping some water between two glasses, pouring it quickly from one glass to the other several times.

Remember I pointed out that a reverse osmosis filter system can leave water "dead"? A typical reverse osmosis unit outputs water with a pH range of 5.2 to 6.4—acidic.

Alkalised water—which is water as it should be in its natural state—is much more readily absorbed by the body, all the way down to the cellular level. That helps boost your metabolism and improves your absorption of nutrients. Effectively, everything about your body works better.

The downside of these systems is cost—mostly over a thousand pounds—but some companies will let you rent one.

I use an ioniser from the Water Ionizing Company run by Lewis Montague. He is one of the most well-informed people I know about health and well-being and how to avoid cancer.

He is so passionate about helping people; he is one of the few companies that will rent you a machine.

I just wish that option had been available 5 years ago when I parted with my money.

Are you diluting your digestion?

A final note on alkalised water: it is often recommended to avoid drinking it for around half an hour (ideally a full hour) either side of eating, or you may disrupt your digestion. The idea is that you don't want to be adding alkaline water to your stomach acid, thus diluting it. However, there is another viewpoint on this.

Your stomach does not actually bring in its acid until about an hour after you have eaten. This is to give time for your saliva and digestive enzymes to do their work first. So your stomach is an alkaline environment anyway, during its first stage of digestion. In which case having a drink with your meal makes little difference.

I personally prefer to drink very little of anything with a meal. Either way, perhaps the best advice is to drink a good glass of water at least half an hour before your meal. This hits the spot in three ways.

- It reduces your feeling of hunger (often thirst in disguise), so you won't be inclined to overeat.
- It ensures there is spare fluid in your system, so your stomach can produce acid without needing to rob water from elsewhere.
- And it won't dilute either your digestive enzymes or your stomach acid.

If you must drink whilst eating, perhaps make it water that has been filtered rather than alkalised.

How much water, and how often?

For your body to work at its best, it needs to have enough water and good quality water. Otherwise, you are putting a huge strain on every bodily system.

I have already explained ways to make sure that the water you are drinking is the good stuff, but how much is enough and how often should you be taking it in?

Half a fluid ounce of water per pound of body weight per day is a formula widely used. Therefore a person weighing ten stone (140 pounds) needs to be drinking 70 fluid ounces, which equals 2 litres.

Simple—but not easy.

How many people actually know their own exact weight? And who has time (or the means) to measure out their water and keep a tally?

Rise and shine

I recommend you do it like this.

Start your day with a couple of large glasses of warm water. You need it to replace the water you lose through perspiring during the night—as well as the water you lose through your breathing.

The warm water is far more easily absorbed by your body and instantly sets you up for the day ahead.

Gently does it

Apart from first thing in the day, the only time I would recommend drinking a large quantity of water in one go is just after you have been exercising or doing heavy work that makes you perspire.

Throughout the day, you want to be sipping ideally warm but at least room temperature water. To help build the habit, keep a glass of drinking water close at hand, whether at home or at work. Sip from it frequently—and refill it as soon as it becomes empty so that your next sip is ready and waiting for you. The longer you leave your glass empty, the more likely you are to "forget" to fill it.

If you drink too much in one go, you will not be hydrating your body, but just going to the loo more often. It's like pouring a lot of water onto a houseplant that has dried out. All that happens is the water flows through the soil and out the bottom of the pot. But add a little water at a time and it will all stay in the soil and revive the plant.

Anything up to half a litre is fine in one go but above that, you will be visiting the bathroom more frequently.

Meal times

Ideally, you don't want to drink anything during the half hour before you eat, nor for about one hour afterwards, to avoid diluting your digestive enzymes.

What most people don't realise is that you are born with a set number of enzymes and when they run out you won't be absorbing all the nutrients and micro-nutrients that you could be. This explains why children can eat food really quickly and suffer no ill effects. Fifty years later, that same person will likely be suffering and having to eat a lot slower and probably be on some form of medication.

Your enzymes are precious—don't waste them by diluting them or indeed by not chewing your food enough.

Beautiful, healthy, alkalised water. My favourite drink in the whole wide world.

We will return to the acid / alkaline issue when we look at food in Eye Opener 8. But briefly, for now, just as with water for the best health...

- you need to be eating lots more alkalising foods (most fruit and especially vegetables) and holding back on the acidic ones (most foods typical of a Western diet: processed foods, dairy, meat, grains and alcohol).

In Eye Opener 8 we will also be looking at some simple ways you can change the pH of your body and ways of testing it.

KEY ACTION POINTS

- Understand that you are almost certainly dehydrated, and you need to change that to enjoy your best health and vitality.
- By the time it gets to your tap, water has been robbed of the life energy that nature put into it and contains things nature did not add to it.
- At the very least, filter the water you drink, make hot drinks with, and cook with—even the water you wash with—and change the filters regularly.
- Make it your priority to choose and install a suitable system to ionise, alkalise and energise your whole water supply.
- Drink plenty of water first thing in the morning, and after exercise or heavy work that makes you sweat.
- Sip room temperature water throughout the day, in between your meals.
- When you feel peckish between meals, try drinking a glass of water first—it may well be what your body really needs.

Eye Opener 3: See The Light!

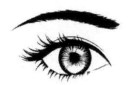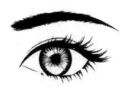

*Also often taken for granted,
sunshine is one of the things,
about which there is
a lot of misinformation.
You will see things
in a new light
after reading this.*

Taking responsibility

Phillip Day inspired my courage to say "no" to conventional treatments and my trust that I instinctively knew what was best for me. His talk at the Grand Hotel in Torquay (when I asked him about radiotherapy), still makes me pause and think, even all these years later. Try this one on for size:

"You are the sum total of all you have ever done to yourself".

Ummm… responsibility for one's own actions. No passing the buck.

He also spoke about the factors that contribute to our immune system allowing cancer to take hold in the body. Factors that we can control. It actually felt good to realise that, if I had helped cause the cancer, then I could also get rid of it and stop it from coming back. Instead of feeling utterly helpless I felt empowered in a way I had never felt before.

We were shown a short animation of life inside a cell. Just one cell out of the trillions that make up our bodies. The information that was imparted that evening was totally life-changing. If you ever get the chance to hear him talk, take it.

What I saw and heard led me to question my view of life as a whole, and the purpose of my own life. At the end of this book, I will revisit spirituality. But for this Eye Opener, I am going to come down to earth and focus on vitamin D—the vitamin that literally does come down to earth: your skin makes it from sunlight.

Ain't no sunshine in my…

I still had some time (after my operation to remove the tumour) before I would be allowed by my doctors to return to full-time work. So I embarked on further research, with vitamin D at the top of my list.

When I was in my mid 20's, there was a lot of publicity about skin cancer and the harmful effects of the sun. So I went from being a dedicated worshipper of the sun to avoiding it like the plague and wearing Sun Protection Factor 15 creams on my face and hands.

In my bid to avoid cancer, I listened to the cancer charities and the government, giving me totally the wrong information. About twenty sun-starved years later, I found myself with cancer—and dangerously low levels of vitamin D.

Enter... Vitamin D

One of the most trusted sources of health information I have found is the world-renowned Dr Mercola. On his website (www.mercola.com) Dr Mercola has an hour-long video presentation (and lots of other articles and videos too) about the huge importance of vitamin D. I urge you to watch it.

Vitamin D is much more than just a vitamin. The body uses it as a hormone and has vitamin D receptors on every cell in your body. Iodine is the only other element that has receptors on every cell. Iodine deficiency is another serious problem and I urge you to read 'The Iodine Crisis' *by Lynne Farrow*. Both play an essential part in hundreds of essential processes (that we know of).

It is known that maintaining optimal vitamin D levels can slash your risk of cancer in half and can prevent many types of cancer altogether—as well as holding at bay a host of other diseases.

What you have to remember is that 90% of what we know about this amazing vitamin has only been discovered in the last decade. You can, therefore, see why this information is not as widely known as it should be. We all need to start educating family and friends about something that could very well save their lives.

On the level

I now have my blood checked on a regular basis to ensure my vitamin D remains at an optimum level.

The UK standard measurement for vitamin D levels is nmol/L—that's nanomoles per litre of blood.

- If you have a major health issue, such as cancer or heart disease, then you want to get your number up somewhere between 175 and 250.

- If you have no major health concerns, then an optimal number is between 125 and 175.
- Below 125, your levels are deficient.
- Above 250, they are in excess.

The most accurate test of how much vitamin D is in your body is the Hydroxy-25 Vitamin D Test. In the UK you can get it via mail order with Birmingham City Assays (www.vitamindtest.org.uk), a department of the NHS Hospitals at Birmingham. They are also able to serve overseas clients.

At the time of writing it costs £28 (UK & Ireland) or £33 + airmail (Overseas). You can call 0121 507 5353 to pay for and order your test kit.

With the test kit, you simply take a couple of drops of blood (which you can easily do yourself) and post it back to them. Within about five working days of receiving your sample, the results are emailed to you.

Check the actual numbers of your test results against the ranges detailed above. Ignore the interpretation on your report of what is considered "adequate", because they use the NHS guideline levels—which are lower, way lower.

Also check carefully, especially if you are getting your test done by a different laboratory, that they are using the same unit of measurement of "nmol/L" (nano-molecules per litre).

All UK labs have been directed to standardise to "nmol/L" but in other countries, labs may still be using the "ng/mL" (nanograms per millilitre) measurement. In which case, multiply by 2.5 to convert to "nmol/L".

So, the next question is, how do we get our vitamin D levels up, and keep them up?

Sunbathing

I now sunbathe every day I can—nothing beats the amazing feel of warm sunshine on my skin. The only thing I avoid is letting my skin burn. Enough exposure to the sun is indicated when the exposed skin is *just about* starting to turn pink. Then it's time to cover up.

The time at which we sunbathe is critical. Vitamin D is not made in our skin every time we sunbathe, only at the time of day when your shadow is shorter than you are. That's around midday.

All the time the sun is shining, we receive UVA rays. They are the ones that give us a tan (and may sometimes trigger skin cancer if we overdo it).

But we only form vitamin D from sunlight when our skin is receiving UVB rays—only present when the sunshine we are getting is at full strength, which is around midday.

We have been told for years to hide from the sun in the middle of the day and only expose ourselves before 11am or after 3pm. Ironically, by doing that we also avoid making vitamin D, which is often found to be deficient in people with skin cancer.

Really, when we are sunbathing to get a tan, that's the time we most need some exposure to the sun at its strongest... so that we get vitamin D from the UVB rays that are only present around midday... to help protect us from the UVA rays that may trigger cancer if we overdo it.

The lies we have been told about sunscreens

Also contrary to the advice we are given, bare skin is the way to go. Most sunscreens contain toxic chemicals. Research has suggested that it is the reaction of these chemicals to sunlight that can trigger cancer. It beggars belief that sunscreens containing these toxins are not only allowed, but recommended.

One last thing to remember—and this is crucial—is that this amazing vitamin is fat soluble and takes up to 48 hours to be made in your skin. If you have a shower and use soap (which contains fat), it will all be washed down the plughole. Shower with just water and use soap if you must, only for your armpits and private parts.

Sunbathing is safe, as long as you take care not to burn and you maintain optimum levels of vitamin D in your body.

As for all the scaremongering about sunshine being the cause of skin cancer, consider these facts and decide for yourself:

- One of the lowest incidences of skin cancer is found among Australian lifeguards, who spend all day exposed to the sun.
- Some of the highest incidences of skin cancer are found amongst office workers in northern countries, who get relatively little sunshine exposure.
- Before the industrial era, when most people lived off the land and spent their time outdoors, skin cancer was rare.
- People with skin cancer are often deficient in vitamin D—which we get from sunshine.
- When skin cancer does appear, it is most often on parts of the body that get least exposure to the sun, such as armpits.

As always, I encourage you to ask questions about everything and check these things out for yourself, if you have the time. But I hope I am saving you a lot of time.

Supplementing

In the UK where I live (even though I'm in the sunniest part of the country, in the South West) it's hard to optimise your vitamin D levels with sun exposure alone. So I take a good quality supplement.

The official recommended daily intake is usually 600 International Units (IU), sometimes as high as 800. But your body uses on average 5,000 IU a day—nearly ten times as much. These recommendations are based on the bare minimum needed to avoid serious disease—not the levels needed for bouncing health. Which would you prefer?

It now turns out that

"Scientists Confirm:
Recommendation for Vitamin D Intake was
Miscalculated and is Far Too Low."

A scientific study completed by UC San Diego and Creighton University says the "miscalculation was by a factor of ten. So, where medical institutes were recommending 600 IU of vitamin D daily for all ages up to seventy (800 for older people), the recommendation should have been around 6,000 IU of vitamin D daily, from all sources.

I knew it!

And that level is still way below the 10,000 IU of vitamin D that is regarded as safe for adults to take in daily.

I personally take 7,000 IU a day, except when I'm getting plenty of sun exposure. Then I don't bother with supplementing. This seems to be what my body needs. Make sure you are supplementing with vitamin D3, not D2. It is D3 that your body needs.

Where you live is important

Unless you live within 50 degrees latitude of the Equator, it is highly unlikely you will be able to get enough sunshine for your skin to convert all the vitamin D that you need. The Tropics are at about half that distance from the Equator. The UK, northern Europe and Canada are just beyond it. Most southern hemisphere countries are within it.

Even then, to get enough vitamin D from sunshine alone, you have to be able to lie outside, naked, for 20 minutes in the noonday sun—assuming that the sun will be shining at noon and not clouded over. And assuming the police don't arrest you before your twenty minutes are up.

So, for most people supplementing is the way to go to get enough vitamin D. Food has such low levels; this is one time you really do have to supplement. The only other option is to use a safe tanning bed. "Safe" means that the ballast (that's the type of resistor coil in the lamp tubes) is an electronic and not a magnetic one.

When supplementing, make sure you are taking vitamin D3. D2 is not the one you need. Also, for Vegans, be aware that D3 is usually made from lanolin, taken from sheep's wool. It is possible to find a vitamin D3 supplement suitable for Vegans (even on Amazon), but you need to check carefully.

There are numerous strengths on the market, so if you have low levels which you probably do, you will need to start off at a higher dose.

My recommendation would be to take 10,000 IU a day

for a month. At this point, I would urge you to get your levels tested, but either way, drop down to 5,000 IU a day.

A word of caution

Nature never works on its own and if using artificial means to raise your levels then consider supplementing with vitamin K2, or eating more fermented vegetables. More about these miracle workers in Chapter Eight.

KEY ACTION POINTS

- Taking care not to burn; enjoy the midday sun whenever you can.
- Ditch the sunscreens—unless you can find one with all-natural ingredients.
- Avoid using soap if you shower after sunbathing.
- Get your vitamin D levels tested.
- Buy a year's supply of vitamin D3 capsules, 5,000 IU strength. The cost will be under £20. Try Amazon if you have no joy with your local shops, but a good Health Food Store will usually have it.
- Assess how much you need to increase by and then decide how you want to do this. I supplement in the winter when I can't sunbathe, but prefer the natural source during summer.

Eye Opener 4: Your Body: Use It or Lose It

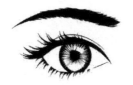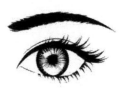

Yes, this means "exercise"…
…but did you know,
the best ways to exercise
are also the easiest?

It isn't all about exercise

Even if you hate exercise and the very mention of the word makes you break out into a cold sweat, please keep reading. This chapter is about movement and that includes down to the cellular level. Keep reading and all will be revealed.

Exercise is simply movement

Your body is designed to move and your health depends on it. You already know that, but even so, did your body just tense up, even a teeny bit, in resistance to the thought of "exercise"?

Well, your body may well be sending you the right message. Even if you are someone who relishes a round at the gym twice a day (and runs there and back), listen up and discover why...

The best ways to exercise are enjoyable—and easy.

Anything you enjoy doing that involves movement counts as exercise—even cleaning the house or pottering in the garden or just shaking it about. As long as you do it regularly. Choosing something enjoyable is the crucial key, otherwise, you won't keep it up regularly.

Enjoyment is an essential factor because, if you are not enjoying the exercise you do, then you are doing it with tension, constricting yourself. Healthy exercise is not so much about pushing your limits (unless you enjoy that). Healthy exercise is more about promoting freedom and flow throughout your body.

Sitting—"the new smoking"

Before we explore the best ways to work out, let's take a look at what happens when we don't exercise, for example, when we are sitting. Nothing much happens, of course, but the trouble is, that includes things that are supposed to be happening to maintain good health.

For example, the heart pumps blood, carrying nutrients and

oxygen to every cell in the body and carrying out waste that needs to be disposed of.

But all that waste can build up and stagnate in your lymphatic system if there is not enough movement in your body to shift it. You see, your lymph is not pumped directly by the heart. It depends on regular, repeated stretching and movement in your body to do the pumping. Without such movement, toxins accumulate.

Of course, we have to sit some of the time, but we were not designed to sit in chairs. Nature designed us to sit by squatting on our haunches. Some chairs are better than others, but most chairs put everything out of proper alignment, which creates undue pressure that strains different internal organs. Eventually, something will give way.

> *Sitting for too long has been described as "the new smoking", for how it adversely affects your health.*

If you have to sit for lengthy periods, such as working at a desk or driving or watching TV, it is important to break it up as much as possible. Research has shown that, for example, an hour at the gym after work, whilst having many benefits, does not really compensate for the ill effects of having sat at a desk all day.

Make sure you get up and stretch and move around every 20 minutes or so. Set a timer if necessary. This really does make all the difference.

Rebounders, those little mini-trampolines that easily fit into the corner of a room (or better still, out in your backyard in the fresh air), are a fantastic, fun way for taking a regular movement break during long spells of sitting.

And something beneficial that you can do even while you are sitting is...

Stretching and yawning

If you don't stretch your muscles regularly, they will over time contract and you will gradually lose your full range of motion.

Watch children at play. See how flexible they are as they

move their bodies. It's a joy to watch. We need not lose any of that freedom of movement.

Getting older does not have to mean getting stiffer.

From the moment you awaken each morning, take every opportunity to stretch. Plus—take a lesson from your dog or cat, if you have one—stretching includes yawning.

Yawning is so contagious; you are probably doing it, or feel like doing it right now, just from reading about it. Let it go, long and wide. Feels good, doesn't it? That's because a yawn releases a dose of your happiness hormones, as well as releasing tension.

Don't worry what others may think—you will be the one behaving naturally, and enjoying the benefits.

For stretching, I personally love Pilates and Yoga and practice both.

Breathing is in the belly...

Another detriment of long sitting and too little movement is shallow breathing. Good exercise invigorates us by giving our lungs a good stretch and getting us breathing more fully—automatically. But it is worth spending some time exploring and adjusting breathing habits.

The muscle designed for breathing is the diaphragm that sits below our lungs, pulling down on them to take a breath in, then releasing to let it out. Not the shoulder muscles trying to heave them up. That means...

If you are breathing the way you are supposed to, your stomach will be moving in and out, and your shoulders will mostly be still.

Apart from nicely massaging your internal organs and stimulating the flow of your digestion, belly breathing ensures that you are drawing breath right down into your lower lungs. That's where most of the blood vessels are, and breathing is all about your blood—exchanging fresh oxygen for waste.

We expel a surprising number of toxins from our bodies

through our breath. As much as 80% of our waste is expelled through the breath. Think about it: you are breathing every moment, day and night, so you might as well get the most benefit from doing it correctly.

If you aren't breathing properly, waste is accumulating in your body and hindering it from working properly. Breathe deeply, as often as you can and make sure your stomach moves with your breathing, not your chest.

...and through your nose

There are many reasons for breathing through your nose, not your mouth—far beyond filtering the air through the fine hairs in your nostrils.

Air coming in through the nose passes through a labyrinth of sinus passages that further filters it, which allows your brain to assess the temperature and humidity and take care of adjusting them to the perfect levels before that air reaches your delicate lungs. If needed the air is warmed by the blood in your nose and breathing out through your nose, in turn, warms up your nose again.

Breathing out through your nose also helps maintain optimum levels of carbon dioxide in your blood. Not all of it is expelled, your body needs to hold onto some of it, but too much carbon dioxide makes your blood more acidic. We saw in Eye Opener Two how that is not good for your health.

I was amazed when I started making the effort to breathe through my nose more. I'd never been a nose breather when exercising. I'd always felt I could not get enough oxygen into my lungs through my nose. Imagine my surprise when, after just one week, I was able to breathe in and out through my nose with ease—AND work out at a faster pace.

But let's begin with something easy...

The walk of life

Endless studies show that a daily walk of twenty minutes—just twenty minutes—is beneficial enough to increase your life expectancy. And that's just normal walking. It need not even be a brisk walk. However, it is a very good idea to make maybe five minutes of any walk brisk. Why? All is revealed when we look at the latest science on exercise.

HIT your workouts

What most people think of first when exercise is mentioned includes things like pounding the treadmill (or pavement) for hours on end. That style of exercise is what's known as "cardio" (cardiovascular). The idea is to get the heart pumping harder, which is not a bad thing to do occasionally.

But it's boring and hard work.

Even the American Heart Association and the American College of Sports Medicine now recognise that long, slow "cardio" is not a good way to optimise your health.

The latest research has shown a far quicker way to get much better results: High-Intensity Interval Training (HIIT). I'll call it HIT. It also goes under the name of Sprint 8 or Peak Eight, PACE, and Tabatha, depending on who you are learning it from, but the same basic principles run through them all.

HIT use the same "cardio" exercises, but in short, intense bursts of around 30 seconds, each followed by a minute or two of easy movement or rest. During those short bursts, you put in 100% effort, followed by recovery, repeating the cycle maybe eight times.

It sounds easy. It isn't. If you are doing them right, HIT is tough. But...

A full HIT workout can be over and done within half an hour. Plus, the health benefits (well documented in numerous studies) are profound. Especially so if you are male. The latest findings show that results aren't as great if you are female—but they are still amazing.

You can apply the principles of HIT to just about any form of exercise that you enjoy doing. For example, if you like running, go for a shorter run overall, but at regular intervals put in a full-pelt spurt followed by a few minutes at an easy pace. The same with cycling, or rowing.

Walking too, in your "daily twenty minutes", you can put in five rounds of walking as briskly as you possibly can for a minute followed by three minutes at an easy pace. No need to be too particular about the exact timings.

Remember, a daily walk of just twenty minutes—that's only about a mile, for most people—is enough to increase your lifespan. Why stop at once a day?

Strength Training

Muscle strength is important to maintain, especially as you get older. Your body is going to have to keep working for you throughout your life. You don't have to get weaker as you get older.

YouTube is full of clips of people demonstrating feats of strength well into their seventies, eighties, even nineties. I especially like the one in which a granny at the gym challenges a group of young hunks to match her bench press—and beats them with ease. It's never too late. Many of these people did not start training until they were past sixty.

To build muscle strength, you simply have to use your muscles on a regular basis. Forget complicated systems that claim to isolate and work particular muscles. The fact is, despite all the fancy names for "different" muscles in the anatomy books, all of your muscles work together as one system. And that's the way nature intends for you to use them.

Some people love going to the Gym to work out their muscles, and that's fine, it can be a social thing, but you can get just as good, if not better results by doing some manual work, such as cleaning your house or gardening. Pick something you enjoy doing, or at least find a way to make it more fun.

If weight training appeals to you, baked bean tins or bags of rocks can be just as effective as any expensive equipment. Don't make excuses, but do make enjoyment of exercise a part of your daily routine.

The perfect plan

So, there you have it, the perfect exercise plan:

- stretching and yawning;
- moving around more;
- breathing with your stomach and your nose;

- short but regular walks;
- a little bit of a workout;
- plenty of what you enjoy doing.

Is any of that difficult?

No fretting about sweating

Has just reading about exercise made you break out in a sweat yet? Of course, sweating is a great part of any exercise routine that enables your body to throw out some toxins. The more often you can sweat, the better. Just make sure you shower the released toxins away before they dry on your skin and get reabsorbed.

You can also sweat while relaxing—in a sauna. In traditional saunas' the air is heated, which then heats your body. Infra-red saunas are more efficient. The infra-red heat goes directly to your body, none being wasted heating the air. The harmless rays also penetrate a few millimetres into your skin, helping the detox process.

Infra-red saunas are more comfortable, to both your body and your wallet than traditional saunas and they are available as portable units or as blankets that you wrap yourself in.

There are many more things you can do, besides working up a sweat, to help your body eliminate toxins.

Now skin yourself

Dry skin brushing is such a simple way to start your day before you shower.

Your skin is the largest detoxifying organ you have. For it to work at its best, the pores need to be cleared of any dead skin cells which clog them up.

Dry skin brushing is a quick, effective way of not only removing those dead skin cells but also stimulating the flow of your lymphatic system (which clears away toxins internally).

All you need is a natural bristle brush and around five minutes.

Start at the soles of your feet and use sweeping strokes to brush your skin, working towards your heart. Work your way up each leg, over your stomach, as much of your back as you can reach, followed by your hands, arms and shoulders—always brushing towards your heart. Stop at the neck area and above.

Then, simply shower off those dead skin cells with your filtered water.

Hot and Cold Showering

Detox happens naturally when the natural movement within your body systems is flowing freely. A quick and simple way to help with this is to alternate the temperature of the water as you shower. Ideally, three one-minute blasts of cold, each followed by a blast of hot. And always finish off with a cold rinse, for maximum refreshment.

Check first that the temperature control on the shower you will be using responds accurately. Do not try this in a shower with a temperature control that is erratic—or you may risk scalding yourself.

What happens is that your body responds to the hot and cold as it naturally tries to regulate its own temperature. During each cold blast, your body takes its blood vessels deeper into itself, to conserve body heat. So during each hot blast, your blood vessels move back to the surface, to throw off excess heat. Thus, you get a "pumping" effect as the blood vessels move inwards and outwards several times, this then pumps the flow of your lymph, which carries away wastes and toxins for elimination.

Simple.

I resisted trying this for a long time but found that it feels so good afterwards, I now can't wait to get in that shower each morning for a round of hot and cold. The actual experience is far less uncomfortable than the initial thought of it.

Oil Pulling

Oil pulling is an age-old remedy that uses natural substances to clean teeth and gums. It has the added effect of whitening teeth naturally, and evidence shows that it is beneficial in improving gum health and removing harmful bacteria.

I discovered oil pulling after my dentist, to my horror, told me I had periodontal disease. He wanted to take x-rays, give me strong antibiotics and deep clean the gums over several weeks—with injections each time. I really didn't want any of that, but nor did I want to have diseased gums sending toxins coursing around my body.

One thing I've learned over recent years is to never do anything out of fear but to do lots of research first.

I went away and decided to give myself six weeks to find a better way. I could still come back to my dentist's plan if nothing else worked.

Oil pulling seemed the obvious choice. It was something I had done for a few months a couple of years previously. I'm not sure why I stopped.

Oil pulling is an ancient practice that has many health benefits, the main one being an improvement in the health of your gums—in fact, your whole mouth benefits. It literally "pulls" out anything that shouldn't be there, including bad bacteria.

It's very easy to do.

First thing each morning, before you do anything else, start by putting a tablespoon of oil into your mouth. Coconut oil is my preferred choice: it has the most amazing anti-bacterial, anti-fungal and anti-microbial properties.

Swish the oil round and round in your mouth, and suck it through your teeth, for about twenty minutes, taking care not to swallow any of it: the oil will be absorbing all the 'nasties' that are in your mouth. After twenty minutes, you spit it all out and give your mouth a thorough rinse. Then clean your teeth as you normally do.

During the twenty minutes, you can be doing other things at the same time. You can also do oil pulling at any time, but it needs to be four hours after eating. I did it twice a day for six weeks; though in hindsight I would say that once a day is fine.

After those six weeks, I went back to my dentist. He told me I no longer needed any treatment—I had cured myself. He recommended returning in three months to check again. I have been back many times now and there is never a problem. On the most recent visit to my dentist, he didn't even need to do a scale and polish.

Oil pulling is now part of my morning ritual. I don't even think about it.

Enemas and colonic cleansing

Ideally, you should be having a bowel movement at least once a day. Some lucky people go more often, but what may be normal for one person isn't necessarily so for another.

The first step to normal elimination is to ensure you are eating plenty of vegetables. I generally eat ten or so portions of vegetables and a couple of fruit each day. That ensures enough fibre to keep things moving.

If waste matter sits in the colon for too long, the toxins waiting to be expelled end up being re-absorbed. So never ignore a call of nature.

Should you need a helping hand occasionally, then enema's (which can be self-administered) can work wonders.

Colonics cleanse the colon much more thoroughly but need to be administered by a practitioner who knows what they are doing. Afterwards, the whole body, and your mind too, feels clean.

So, there you have a few fun things you can do, as well as exercise and build up a sweat, to help your body eliminate toxins. In the next Eye Opener, we take a look at how lots of unnatural chemical toxins get into our bodies in the first place—and how we can easily stop their invasion.

KEY ACTION POINTS

- Minimise the time you spend sitting and break it up with frequent stretching and moving around.
- Learn to breathe more slowly and more deeply, using your belly and your nose.
- Whenever it's an option, walk. Also, take the stairs rather than the lift.
- Say goodbye to long and boring exercise. Go for short, intense bursts of whatever you do.
- Find something you can enjoy doing regularly that keeps

your muscles working.

- Consider getting an infra-red sauna.
- Dry brush your skin before your morning shower.
- Tone yourself up with "hot and cold" showers.
- Try oil pulling for healthy teeth and gums.
- Consider occasional enemas and colonics to keep clean internally.

Eye Opener 5: Clean Up Your Cleaning

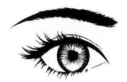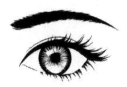

*Keeping things clean
could actually be polluting your body
and slowly killing you.
Here's how to really clean up,
without compromising
your health.*

Home sweet home?

Most homes are a minefield of toxic chemicals and heavy metals. Even the briefest contact with your skin provides them with a very short step to get into your body—and they will.

However much or often you try to detox your body, you are fighting a losing battle unless you also take a careful look at the chemical cocktails you are exposing yourself to in the home—and do something about it.

Wearing rubber gloves is not enough to protect you from the health hazards in household cleaning products. They leave residues everywhere and get into the air you breathe. The only safe place for them is to leave them on the supermarket shelves and not allow them into your home at all.

Besides protecting your health, cleaning up your cleaning will also save you money. Because you can get just as good results, probably even better, with traditional natural cleansing agents such as baking soda, cider vinegar and lemon juice. You won't find "DO NOT SWALLOW" labels on any of those.

However, saving you money is just an added bonus. What we are talking about here, is saving your health.

Kitchens and bathrooms

This is where most domestic cleaning goes on. For any surface (including tiles or lino floors and windows) a mixture of bicarbonate of soda and vinegar (white wine vinegar or apple cider vinegar), diluted in water will do the job.

Keep it simple. You don't need hoards of cleaning chemicals.

If you prefer something "ready to use" that you don't need to mix up yourself, try Libby Chan. It's a probiotic cleaner. You can even drink it. Yet it is effective at cleaning your toilet.

Avoid all anti-bacterial products like the plague: they often contain Triclosan. More and more studies are linking Triclosan (and its chemical cousin Triclocarban) to adverse health effects, ranging from skin irritation to endocrine disruption. Rather than wiping out bacteria, they help breed strains resistant to antibiotics.

You don't want that stuff in your home. Nor do you want to even flush it down the drain. Contamination of water has an untold negative impact on the delicate balance of our planet's aquatic ecosystems.

Mould

Speaking of mini eco-systems. One that you do *not* want in your home is mould. It doesn't stay on hidden-away parts of walls and windowsills. It sends spores out into the air. If there is mould anywhere in your home, you are breathing it.

When tackling mould, rubber gloves and a mask are a must, as well as maximum ventilation. After you have scrubbed off as much as you can, wipe down the affected area with slightly diluted apple cider vinegar and repeat the treatment regularly. You will find that the mould takes longer to return—if it does.

Fresh Air?

Real fresh air is just that: fresh air, free from chemical sprays. Be especially wary of room fresheners described as "sea breeze" or "spring fresh"—all they do is trick you with chemicals. The best (and again, the cheapest) way to get real fresh air into your home is to keep windows open as much as possible (day and night).

It may seem counter-intuitive, but even in winter, if you've had windows open all day, you will find that in the evening your home warms up more quickly and feels cosier. That's because good ventilation clears out excess moisture from the air—moisture that you are otherwise paying to heat up.

Laundry and clothes

Most laundry powders and liquids contain toxic chemicals. There is an alternative: natural soap, which is extracted from nuts. But I admit that can be fiddly to use.

I have found an easy alternative in Laundry Eco Eggs. It's well worth looking them up on the internet. Just to give you an idea, using my Eco Egg costs me about £6 for a whole year, and

I use my washing machine around four times a week.

One thing I use it for, and highly recommend, is to wash brand new clothes *before* I wear them for the first time. More and more, clothing fabrics (even natural ones like cotton and wool) are being treated with various chemicals. You don't want toxic chemicals touching your skin in any way.

Personal hygiene and body care

As we have already seen, anything you put on your skin also goes into your body. Ideally, you don't want to put anything on your skin that you wouldn't eat.

Any items containing Sodium Laurel Sulphate, BPA's or perfume should be avoided. You won't find many that don't— even in health stores. I'd advise you to check the ingredients.

These days, what I personally use is…

- Bicarbonate of soda for deodorant.
- Argan oil for my face and body and a natural soap for my sensitive areas.

You really don't want to be using any soap over your body because it removes the protective oil that nature provides.

Make-up and beauty products

How long, on average, do all those bottles and jars sit on your dressing table or bathroom shelf? That's why most of those products are laden with chemical preservatives that should not go anywhere near any part of your body.

For a long time, I thought this was one area I would have to compromise on. Although when I looked, I found that there are many beautiful, non-toxic, affordable ranges on the market. You will be spoilt for choice.

Great ranges that I have tried include Lavera, Lily LoLo, Green People and Benecos. As always, check the label carefully.

Heavy metal

I'm not talking Ozzy Osbourne here. Even in his wildest days, he was a pussycat compared to the health threat posed by heavy metals of the chemical variety.

More and more, heavy metals are getting into the food chain, a major source being the industrial pollution pouring into the air, into the oceans and into the soils of the earth. As well as being absorbed into crops, tiny creatures cannot help but ingest them. These are, in turn, eaten by bigger creatures... and end up in the food on our plates.

It makes sense to avoid anything originating from countries with fewer controls over industrial pollution, such as China. That's another thing—country of origin—to check carefully on food labels, besides the actual ingredients.

Mike Adams, "the health ranger" from Natural News, has spent year's thoroughly investigating levels of heavy metals in foods. His website (www.naturalnews.com) is well worth looking at for more information on this.

On a brighter note, here are three ways you can protect yourself from heavy metals hidden in food.

- Strawberries help stop heavy metals being absorbed. Just be sure they are organic. You'll see why at the 'Dirty Dozen' list in my final Eye Opener.
- Chlorella (a green algae) is excellent for helping to detox your body and remove harmful substances. Sprinkle it on salads or into your green smoothies.
- Likewise, coriander leaf (cilantro) is an excellent helper in removing toxic metals from your body.

Furniture and Soft Coverings

Legislation on Fire Regulations now ensures that most household soft furnishings are treated with toxic chemicals. That includes sofas, beds, carpets, curtains... anything that might potentially go up in flames. A good reason not to replace your old sofa.

Even if you cover the item up, as you do with sheets on your bed, those chemicals are going to "gas" and build up in the air you are breathing.

Here's what you can do about it if you have to buy a new item. Firstly, remove any packaging immediately. If you have anywhere outside of your home where you can keep the furniture, store it there for as long as possible, to give any gases time to dissipate.

When you bring the item into your house, turn up the heating to maximum, close all windows and allow the heat to build. Leave the house. After a few hours return, open all the windows and give the item a good pounding to shake out as much of the chemicals as possible. Wear a mask for that.

You won't get rid of all the chemicals, but you will have minimised their effect. You can minimise it further by making a point of opening windows whenever possible, even if for a short space of time to get a flow of fresh air into your home.

The more time your furniture spends outdoors, the better.

Take your time, but quickly

There are a lot of changes to be made here. It will take time. But the points covered in this Eye Opener are probably the ones people neglect the most. Make it your priority to deal with these things systematically.

Once you start making these changes, they become easier.

KEY ACTION POINTS

- Stop risking your health by using chemicals to clean your home—they are actually polluting it.
- Start finding out about and learning to use safe, natural cleaning agents that really do leave your home fresh and clean. Most household cleaning can be done with baking soda, natural vinegar and lemon juice.
- Keep fresh air flowing through your home as much as possible, and do as much as you can to minimise pollution from new furniture.
- For true personal care, don't put anything on your own body that you would not eat—because you are "eating" it through your skin.
- Start trying out non-toxic make-up made from natural ingredients. As they say in the famous adverts… "You're worth it!"

Eye Opener 6: Are You Short-Circuiting Yourself?

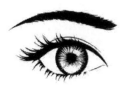 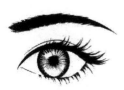

*We are all immersed—
mostly drowning—in a soup
of electro-magnetic fields.
Here's how you can swim
and stay on top.*

Electrical Smog

Virtually all of us take advantage of modern technology and use electrical devices on a daily basis. Very few of us consider what the effects of these electromagnetic fields will have on our health. Part of this is that we have become reliant on them and almost everyone owns a mobile phone and wouldn't consider leaving home without it. These fields can penetrate up to 17cm into the body and have been linked to childhood leukaemia amongst other things. Even fluorescent lights can leave us feeling more tired than we should and not feeling as alert as we would like to be. The lethargy we feel is a result of our red blood cells clumping together when exposed to these concentrated electromagnetic fields.

How many devices do you own?

Have a think about all the electrical devices you are exposed to every day. Scary. Even electric clock radios emit relatively high electromagnetic fields, so having these on your bedside table isn't a good idea at all. Anything which requires electricity to work will emit a level of electromagnetic field around it.

Do you live near overhead power lines?

A study undertaken by Dr Nancy Wertheimer showed that when children live close to overhead power lines they are 3 times more likely to develop cancer and leukaemia than children who live a safe distance away. A safe distance to live from these power lines is estimated to be a minimum of a fifth of a mile away. Where is your closet line?

Medical equipment—friend or foe?

Even our medical equipment designed to improve our health exposes us to unnecessarily high levels of electromagnetic fields and radiation. X-rays and so-called diagnostic scans are just some examples. Mammograms are a big one that springs to mind. I won't ever have another one and it has nothing to do with squishing my breasts between two metal plates and then putting radiation through them.

Umm, can that really be healthy?

The Mammogram I had when I found my lump was exceptionally painful and it didn't even pick up a problem.

A safer alternative

Thermograms offer a safe alternative and one that I use each year to ensure I am still on track. The pictures below show the progress I made by changing my diet and lifestyle over a relatively short space of time.

The cancer was in my right breast. The first picture was taken 5 months after the surgery and around 7 months into the changes I was beginning to make. Picture two was taken another 3 months later. More improvements can be seen and then in the third picture around 21 months after the operation you can clearly see the improvement in the health of my breasts. By then I had changed a lot of things in my life and they all had had a chance to heal my body.

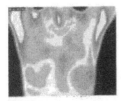
February 2010

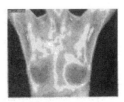
May 2010

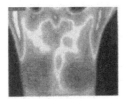
June 2011

Do you suffer from any of these?

Other conditions which may be caused by exposure to electromagnetic fields are severe headaches, fatigue, brain cancer and tumours, memory and concentration problems, nausea, nervous system damage, tinnitus, sleeplessness, asthma, allergies, arthritis, weakened immune systems, epilepsy, Alzheimer's, strokes, heart attacks, severe cases of exhaustion, birth defects and even miscarriages. The list goes on as we find out more.

A healthy balance

I have made a number of changes that I am happy with and feel that there has to be compromise with enjoying the many benefits of technology and protecting yourself as much as possible. Admittedly when I first found out about EMF's, early on in my journey, I immediately got rid of my cordless phones (much to the annoyance of my two teenage children) and bought a long extension lead. I still won't allow a cordless phone in the house, even a number of years later, although I understand that you can buy ones that aren't as harmful to you. I turned off my Wi-Fi and used Ethernet power adapters, which are devices that use your electrical wiring to transfer the internet to your device.

Now with my partner and his two children refusing to not have Wi-Fi, I comprise and use the Ethernet adapters in the daytime when I am working from home and just use the Wi-Fi for a few hours in the evening. Even if you aren't convinced about the potentially harmful effects of electromagnetic fields it can't do any harm to turn off your wireless router at night, can it? If you think you might forget then buy a cheap timer so that it automatically switches it off for you. When you are sleeping and your cells are repairing and doing what cells do, it has to be a good idea to allow them to have the best possible conditions. We are after all electrical beings.

Staying safe while mobile

Mobile phone harmful effects can be reduced by not carrying it near your body and when you are using the phone for calls use the speaker function whenever you can. A number of ladies have started carrying their devices in their bra strap and as a result, a number of cancerous tumours have been discovered in the same shape as the phone. Scary.

So keep your phone away from your body. Even the instructions that come with your phone will tell you to keep it away from the body. Have a read of your instruction manual, if you don't believe me. Turn it off at night, put it onto flight mode, or at the very least move it to another part of your home.

In an ideal world I would like to have a switch inside my home to cut all power to the house overnight, however, my family members would all probably leave home and I would hate that.

Other ways to protect yourself

You can buy special paints for your walls to protect yourself and drapes you can sleep under but they are expensive. A cheaper alternative is a grounding sheet for your bed. Clinton Ober has written a fabulous book called 'Earthing: The Most Important Health Discovery Ever?' In the book, he explains in detail how important it is to literally ground ourselves with the earth. There are many other devices you can buy to help ground you and a great one is a mat you rest your feet on when using electrical devices.

There are safety measures that you can take to help reduce your exposure to electromagnetic fields. Consider unplugging and turning off all electrical appliances when they are not being used, take breaks when you might have to work for prolonged times on computers and TVs, keeping all electrical appliances at least 6 feet away from your bed, moving your mobile phone to another room at night or even turning it off, and using electrical appliances for as brief periods as possible. Walk barefoot outside on grass or sand for 20 minutes a day if possible.

Indoor plants can be very beneficial because they are able to absorb some of the fields and radiation whilst at the same time producing negative ions which are necessary for our bodies. They look beautiful too.

KEY ACTION POINTS

- Consider if you need that medical diagnostic test or is there a safer one you could use.
- Go back to corded phones or at least move the base station away from the bedroom.
- Turn off your wireless router whilst you are asleep—you don't need it then.
- Keep your mobile phone away from your body and use the speakerphone when possible.
- Text instead of talking on your mobile.
- Consider using protective paints when you redecorate your home.
- Take regular breaks when using electrical devices, at least every 30 minutes as a minimum.
- Unplug devices from the wall when not using them.
- Try barefoot walking, ideally on damp grass or sand.
- Buy some beautiful indoor plants.

Eye Opener 7: Mind Your Stress

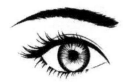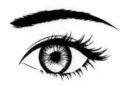

Stress is recognised as
a major cause of
much physical illness—
but it often begins with
our thoughts and feelings.
Here's how to get away
and stay away from stress.

Phillip Day's Insight

When I went to Phillip Day's talk at the Grand Hotel back in 2009 I have no doubt that it was a major turning point in my life. If you haven't read his books or watched his free films then I urge you to. He is my guru and I aspire to have his values and knowledge. He is "The Man!"

Phillip is an investigative journalist who travels the country and the world giving talks on the real reason we are all getting sicker and offering ways for people to take control of your own health.

During the interval, I went and spoke to him about the cancer I had had and one of the things he said to me was that I must be very stressed.

I laughed and said

"No, I have a stress free life".

His reply was something along the lines of "most ladies who get breast cancer have a lot of stress in their lives and I should really sort it out if I wanted to prevent the cancer from returning."

In hindsight, I can see very clearly where I was going wrong although at the time, being immersed in the situation I couldn't see the wood for the trees.

Delving deeper into the causes

My uncle, Graham Booth was a man I very much admired because he stood up for his views and wanted to make a difference to the world. He had already had one successful career in the hotel and catering industry but that wasn't enough for him.

He had very strong views on the European Union and all it stood for and this made him stand and become an MEP for the South West of England.

He did this for a number of years but finally wanted to retire and enjoy his time with Pam, his wife. We spoke one evening and he asked if I would consider standing in the forthcoming election. Wow. Scary stuff, but I too was passionate about the powers we had given away and I thought I too might be able to make a difference. I said "Yes" and threw myself into learning facts and making public speeches.

The stress builds

As time went along I was becoming more and more uncomfortable with the role I had found myself in and could see no way out. I didn't want to disappoint my uncle by standing down and so carried on doing something I didn't want to. That stress, I am sure had a massive effect on me and certainly had an impact on the cancer developing. It wasn't only the situation I was in but many other contributing factors that caused the cancer to grow. The way I was preparing my food, what food I was eating and the cooking processes, plus many other things covered in this book, all had an effect I am sure.

The perfect excuse

When I was diagnosed with breast cancer a few months later I was given the perfect excuse to stop. The Universe answers your requests in very strange ways. So be very careful what you wish for.

I had already decided that I would do virtually anything that might help me on my road to recovery and even though I didn't think I was stressed I embarked on another exploration—to discover new ways to treat stress.

Various tools to try

Meditation is the one that I started with and to be truthful I did struggle in the beginning. How could my mind ever be still when I had so much to think about and learn? I am sure if you have ever tried to meditate you will at some point have had the same experience.

My 5-minute trick

It was at this point I realised that little and often is the key and I would sit down quietly twice a day and I would tell myself I only had to try and still my mind for 5 minutes and then I could go back to what I was doing before. A perfect example of me being stressed and not realising it.

Gradually over time, the 5 minutes grew longer and I would easily find 10 or 15 minutes had gone by. I learnt that I could just watch the thoughts like little clouds but not link any particular emotion to them. It really can be that easy. You can turn your concentration over to your breathing which often helps quieten the chatter or repeat a mantra over and over again.

What is important is that you do it regularly and I find having a little ritual helps me. For me I sit or lie, depending on what I am trying to achieve, I close my eyes and take 2 deep breaths in through my nose and out through my mouth. I have done this so many times now, my body instantly realises that I am in meditation mode and my thoughts calm down. When your mind slows down you can experience flashes of inspiration. The idea of creating a website was just one of those sparks that happened to me, as was leaving my very secure job of 10 years and setting up my company Get Seriously Healthy.

Mindfulness

There are many ways to meditate, but I wouldn't recommend you get too involved in the various techniques to start with. Mindfulness can be done throughout your day and certainly makes the phrase "living in the moment" take on a whole new meaning but the aim of this book is to make any changes easy and quick and what could be more simple than closing your eyes, being aware of your breathing and relaxing for 5 minutes, a couple of times a day?

Meditation can help reduce and even eliminate stress but it is just as important to try to stop it from happening in the first place and the way you view the things that happen to you needs to be addressed.

Half full?

Now is your glass half full or half empty? Are you an optimist or a pessimist? The pessimists of this world often give up at this point because they feel they can't change something that is a part of who they are and how they view the world. I want to tell you that you *can,* and it can be surprisingly easy to do. Keep reading you pessimists.

A Complaint Free World

I have always been an optimist but there is always room for improvement and so I started to look at ways to make me more optimistic, especially about my health. Will Bowen has written a fabulous book called 'A Complaint Free World' and I would recommend you read it. One of the tips he suggests you do is to put an elastic band on your wrist and every time you complain or say something negative you move the band from one wrist to another. This normally happens 30 or 40 times or even more a day, but very quickly you can drop down to moving it just once every 4 or 5 days. Taking the whole challenge to go 21 days can take much longer and a friend of mine took 6 months, but he did it.

Recognising the symptoms

There are many other things you can do to reduce stress but the first thing you need to do is recognise the symptoms. It took me a long time until somebody told me to imagine a really stressful situation and feel where in my body it felt different to normal. By doing this simple exercise I realised that the excited feeling I often had in my tummy wasn't a good feeling at all, but the direct result of stress. That simple tip has changed my life and when that feeling starts I can take steps to reduce the stress.

This is where mindfulness comes in. As soon as I get the feeling, and it does get easier to recognise it, the more you practise, I imagine myself stepping out of my body and watching what I am doing. More as an observer than a participant is the easiest way of explaining it.

Your little voice

We all have an inner voice and can have interesting conversations when it is urging us to do something. Have you ever found your inner voice being quite cruel to you? Now would you allow that dialogue to go on with your best friend with the same tone or words? I would like to think you would immediately say "NO!" Well, by standing back and observing a situation that you find yourself in, you tend to be kinder and gentler on yourself. This really does work but you need to remember to do it when in a situation. The old adage "practise, practise, practise" springs to mind.

Emotional Freedom Technique

The Tapping Solution or EFT is a very simple, free and effective way of helping you in many areas of your life, both physical and mental. Although the actual technique is quite new, the science behind it is thousands of years old. EFT is based on the subtle energy system of acupuncture meridians.

Books have been written on the subject but very briefly you repeat statements whilst at the same time tapping on certain points on your body, mainly the head. The results are profound and can be life-changing.

The technique

To begin you need to assess on a scale of 1 – 10 how bad the situation is making you feel. It is usually a high number.

Start by using the fingers of one hand to tap the side of your other hand below your little finger. This is called the Karate Chop. Repeat 3 times as you are tapping the Karate Chop

"Even though I .... (insert your problem, such as "I am stressed"), I deeply and completely love and accept myself".

You then say a phrase using words relating to the problem as you tap each of the nine points. Please see the picture of me and the points to tap on the next page.

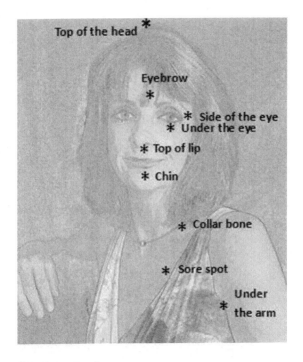

Tapping Points

If you have problems sleeping, for instance, you might say the following.

"I worry about not sleeping" as you tap the eyebrow point.

"I am concerned my body is not repairing properly" as you tap the side of the eye.

"I hate not being at my best because I can't concentrate" as you tap under the eye.

"I will not perform very well" as you tap your upper lip.

"Help! I need to get 8 hours sleep" as you tap your chin.

"My immune system will be weakened" as you tap your collarbone.

"I need more sleep" as you tap the sore point.

"I am worried about my health" as you tap in your armpit.

Finish the round by tapping the top of your head as you

say a final phrase, such as "I hate the worry of not sleeping properly".

Repeat the process 3 times becoming more positive each round, making sure the final set is all in the positive.

Now reassess on a scale of 1 – 10 how you feel about the situation. It should have decreased significantly.

There are many variations on the technique and you can use it for almost any situation or ailment. I used it to help my breathing a year or so after the cancer was discovered. My chest never felt fully expanded and I couldn't take a really deep breath. Apparently, this is a normal "side effect" of having had cancer but one round of EFT and I could breathe again easily. Powerful stuff.

Needless to say, I am a big fan now and recommend this technique to lots of people. It isn't often you come across something that is free, quick, easy and works.

My final suggestion is making sure you have time for yourself each day to do the things that truly make you happy. It might be going for a brisk walk, a bike ride, eating a bar of exceptionally high-quality chocolate, reading a book on the sofa or just talking to a friend. It doesn't matter what it is, just make sure you do more of the things that make you happy. After all, you can't make others happy if you aren't happy yourself.

KEY ACTION POINTS

- Identify what might be causing you to become stressed and if possible remove the cause.
- Learn to meditate on a daily basis even if it is for 5 minutes.
- Explore other techniques that might work better for you. Google is always a good place to start.
- Watch somebody practising the Emotional Freedom Technique on YouTube and see the profound effects it can have. Even better, why not have a go yourself?
- Take more time each day to do the things that bring joy into your life.

Eye Opener 8: Eat Slow To Glow

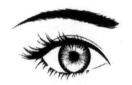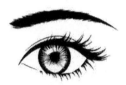

"You are what you eat"
Right?
No. You can only be
what you digest.
Here's how to ensure gut health,
the master key to overall health.

JULIE HARRISON

I am sure you have heard the saying:

"You are what you eat"

This is partly true but really you are what you absorb from the food you eat. You could be eating the best nutritious food in the world and not absorbing it. What a waste.

The processed truth

What you put into your body is ultimately reflected back to you by how your body looks and feels. Processed foods, including all packaged and tinned products, should be eliminated and meals made from scratch. I can almost feel you quivering. Making a quick, beautiful meal from a few basic store cupboard ingredients should take you no longer than 20 minutes and if you are clever and make more than you need you have got lunch covered or dinner the following evening. Don't make things hard for yourself. The secret is to know where to spend your time and money and when to save it.

Check out my recipe book, 'Deliciously Healthy', for some great additions to your repertoire.

If there is an ingredient listing on a product try and give it a wide berth, but at a bare minimum at least know what they all mean and the effect they have on your body.

Sugar isn't so sweet after all

Sugar is an evil substance and should be avoided wherever possible, especially refined sugar. Unrefined sugar is still sugar, as are all the so-called healthy alternatives, such as agave, rice syrup, honey and maple syrup. Yes, you are getting added nutrients but nothing you can't get from a vegetable. I used to believe it was just empty calories that would rot my teeth but I now understand what it actually does to the body. We get quite enough glucose from everything else we eat.

Dr Robert Lustig has a fabulous lecture on 'YouTube', called 'Sugar The Bitter Truth' explaining in more detail how we have been hoodwinked over the years about sugar.

Organic is best, but do you want better?

Eating organically is obviously the way to go, but it can be expensive and you need to make sure you are making your money work well for you. Each year a Dirty Dozen and Clean Fifteen lists are produced by the Environmental Working Group, which has the 12 fruits and vegetables that are most contaminated with pesticides and the 15 least contaminated.

If you eat organically from the most contaminated list and save money by eating conventionally grown items on the Clean Fifteen List then you can reduce your toxic load by around 75%. Now doesn't that sound like a really useful list? The following are lists produced for 2015 but if you are reading this after then you might want to check out http://www.ewg.org to see if there are any changes.

The Dirty Dozen are apples, celery, cherry tomatoes, cucumber, grapes, nectarines, peaches, potatoes, sugar snap peas, spinach, strawberries and peppers.

The least contaminated or the Clean Fifteen are asparaguses, avocados, cabbage, cantaloupe melon, cauliflower, aubergine, grapefruit, kiwi, mangoes, onions, papayas, pineapples, sweet corn, frozen peas and sweet potatoes.

The items on the Clean Fifteen list have relatively low levels of pesticides so if you are trying to save money buy these items. However, nothing can compare to organically grown vegetables and fruit, both nutritionally and in taste, as well as the impact on this wonderful planet we live on. It is always worth checking prices because sometimes organic produce is the same price as conventionally grown items, and sometimes even cheaper. Always check.

Bio-dynamic farming

Growing crops in harmony with nature and the moon's cycle make for far more health-enhancing food. You can easily use some of the principles yourself when growing your own sprouted seeds. Or to have the optimum combination, grow as much of your own food as possible. There is nothing in the world like picking some salad leaves and eating them within a few minutes. Talk about being fresh.

Carnivore or Herbivore?

If you eat meat and animal products you need to ensure that they are raised to organic standards and fed a natural diet with lots of grass.

Conventional farming produces meat which is unhealthy for many reasons. The animals get sicker much more frequently and so their need for antibiotics is greater, which means you develop resistance to them and they might not work when you need them to.

For a number of months, I followed a vegan diet to give my body a chance to recover but I started to crave meat and so introduced a small amount but ensuring it was grass-fed and raised to the highest of standards.

Animal Feed—GMO?

Unless the animals are raised to organic standards you have no control over the type of feed they are having and genetically modified feed is common practice.

I urge you to gather more information to start making informed decisions yourself. Eating better quality meat but in smaller portions is better for you and the planet on so many levels. Also, don't overlook offal as a nutrient-dense food with a very low price tag.

In times gone by...

Hundreds of years ago we all led much more active lives and eating 4,000 odd calories a day was not uncommon. Combine this with how rich and fertile the soil was and it is easy to see with our calorie intake reduced by half and our depleted soils, we are becoming deficient in many vitamins but especially minerals.

Supplementing is almost a necessity

Unless you are eating your own home grown food and making your meals from basic ingredients, avoiding all processed foods there is every chance you will need to supplement your diet. There is no one size fits all, although some brands come close.

Ideally, you want your supplements to be whole food or food-based so your body recognises them as food and not something foreign. You need to research the companies you give your money to so that you can ensure you are happy with the quality of what they are selling as well as their ethical status. You might want to check out whether they have any ties to the big pharmaceutical companies.

A really high-quality multivitamin and mineral supplement is a good starting point. Add in krill oil and some magnesium transdermal spray plus 5,000 IU of vitamin D3 together with iodine and you are covering a lot of deficiencies.

There are a number of supplements which help to detoxify your body which almost everyone needs to do while living in our modern world, with Chlorella being the most widely used. Always start off with a small dose and increase gradually to avoid any potential detoxification problems.

Get organised in the kitchen

The secret to producing near effortless, delicious, nutritious and economical meals is to get organised.

I can almost feel your fear. Trust me, I have had decades of experience and pride myself on doing just that. By having a store cupboard full of essential ingredients, a fridge with a few basics, a freezer stocked with some considered purchases and your new routine and you will be able to produce wonderful food in super quick time.

Juicing versus Smoothies? Now there is a question

So much is spoken about juicing and there is no denying it

can have a profound effect on your health. A juice detox for a few days can be a fantastic kick-start to get you motivated and seeing results fast. An excellent film to watch is 'Fat, Sick and Nearly Dead', if you feel the need to be inspired. I am often asked which is best. There is no right answer and it all depends on what you are trying to achieve.

Types of juicers

There are many different types of juicers with the noisy centrifugal juicers being the cheapest. The juice gets aerated and so will spoil more quickly than the macerating juicers, which although quieter are larger and a little more difficult to clean.

Luckily technology has improved and the latest vertical slow juicers, although more expensive, are exceptionally quiet in operation, the juice doesn't separate and it has a higher nutritional value.

Beautiful vegetables

When you first start juicing you will probably concentrate on fruit juices but these interfere with your insulin resistance and should be avoided. You need to be juicing lots of beautiful vegetables and limiting your fruit. A good tip is to gradually reduce the fruit whilst at the same time increasing the vegetables used. Lemon or lime juice added to a green juice helps to take away the bitterness.

A simple carrot, beetroot, cucumber, celery and kale juice is divine. Maybe consider adding some apple or pineapple to sweeten it, although avoid if you can. The aim is to get drinking green juices as much as possible.

Jason Vale has written some excellent books that go into lots of detail and he has some wonderful recipes.

Smoothies

There is no denying that juicing can be expensive and some people hate the idea of wasting the pulp. There is an alternative. Smoothies are a great way to up your nutritional intake and are so quick and easy to make. You can add in all sorts of superfoods—Maca, Spirulina, Chlorella, bee pollen, goji berries, chia seeds and of course nuts. The basic starting point is to add some greens such as spinach, fruit such as a banana to make it creamy, possibly some berries, nut milk or water if you are adding nuts. Blitz in a food processor, ideally a high-speed one like a Vitamix, but any will do. No wastage and the jug of the blender will take just seconds to clean.

Breakfast like a King?

This is the one meal I used to struggle with when I made my changes. In the years BC (before cancer) I would often have a slice of toast with butter and marmalade or bran flakes or something similar. I remember for months trying to find alternatives. Now it is the easiest meal of all. Why not try a vegetable juice or smoothie, chia porridge (my favourite) or even some roasted vegetables with a softly poached egg. Chia porridge is made with a couple of tablespoons of chia seeds, a mixture of chopped nuts, seeds, Maca powder, berries and optional bananas. Add almond milk and either make the night before and leave in the fridge or leave to thicken for 10 minutes or so.

Lunchtime suggestions

Now I have discovered fermented vegetables (covered at the end of this eye opener), lunch is a dream to make. I usually have 4 or 5 different varieties in the fridge so I never get bored with the flavours.

Depending on what is in season and the time of year lunch might be a vegetable soup or stew in the depths of winter or a bowl of fermented vegetables, salad and either hummus, boiled egg, guacamole or a sandwich made with toasted spelt sourdough bread filled with avocado, grated carrot, beetroot, red onion, salad leaves, homemade mayonnaise and tomato. If you have any leftovers from dinner the night before you can easily dress them up and create another meal in seconds. Forget using a microwave—all you need to do to heat your meals is to add a little water to a pan and gently warm through on the hob.

Dinner anyone?

I adore spicy foods as much as traditional recipes and love to experiment and take meals up a few nutritional notches. It really can be as easy as swapping your intensively reared meat to organic grass-fed meat and increasing your vegetable intake purchasing organic or from the Dirty Dozen list. Swap the vegetable oils for coconut oil and try not to use high heat for your cooking. Add in a beautiful salad to up your raw food and possibly some fermented vegetables and you have already made some changes that your body will love you for.

Ingredients to Swap

When you decide you want to improve your health you often want to find alternatives. I certainly did. However, my choices weren't always great and indeed some of them were worse than the products I was replacing

This is my list of things you can start with by swapping:

- Margarine for organic grass fed butter.
- Butter for coconut oil.
- Vegetable oil for coconut oil.
- Rice for buckwheat, quinoa or chopped raw cauliflower.
- Pasta for courgettes.
- White sugar for Rapadura, or ideally Stevia.
- Coffee for herbal teas.
- Fizzy drinks for sparkling mineral water or unpasteurised homemade juice.
- Cow's milk for coconut, oat or almond milk.
- Table salt for Himalayan Rock salt.
- Wheat flour for spelt, buckwheat or gram flour.
- Tinned tomatoes for glass jars of passata.
- Crisps for home roasted nuts or kale chips or popcorn.
- Cheese for nutritional yeast in recipes.
- Sweets for goji berries and dried mulberries.

- Tuna for sardines, remove skin and bones if necessary.
- Shop bought mayonnaise for super healthy homemade mayonnaise.
- Jams for preserves that use fruit juice instead of sugar.

Your gut health and why it is so important

90% of the genetic material in your body is not your own. Our cells are outnumbered by microbial ones by 100 to 1. Before you become too horrified and reach for the antibacterial wipes and sprays, consider your microflora (which is made up of bacteria, fungi, viruses and other micro-organisms) influences many parts of who you are. Such as your

- genetic expression;
- immune system—80%is based in the gut;
- what you weigh;
- risk of numerous chronic and acute diseases—including intolerances; and
- even your mental health.

Did you know that you actually have two nervous systems?

Your central nervous system which is composed of your brain and spinal cord, which is the one everyone knows about and your enteric nervous system, which is the intrinsic nervous system of your gastrointestinal tract.

Both are actually created out of the same type of tissue. The systems are connected via the vagus nerve with your gut actually sending far more information to your brain than your brain sends to your gut.

Fermenting your foods

By including fermented foods into your diet you are enhancing the nutritional value of foods by increasing B vitamins, vitamin C and some K2. You are also helping your body to detoxify because the beneficial bacteria in these foods are highly potent detoxifiers, capable of drawing out a wide range of toxins and heavy metals.

Saving you money

Fermented foods are also extremely cost-effective. By adding just a small amount of fermented food to each meal will give you the biggest value for your money. Why?

Because they can contain 100 times more probiotics than a supplement.

A quick recipe

Fermenting foods is really easy and all you need to do is to cut up some organic cabbage, add a little good quality salt and pound until the juices start to come out of the cabbage. Pack into a glass and press firmly down until the juices cover the cabbage and the little air pockets have gone. Put a weight on top to hold the cabbage under the liquid, cover and leave to ferment for a minimum of one week. At that point, you can store in the fridge. Start off by just including a teaspoon a day and build up to one cup full. There are some wonderful variations to this simple method and I urge you to spend a while on the internet researching further recipes or buy my recipe book, 'Deliciously Healthy'.

Your secret weapon

Nature provides us with wonderful digestive enzymes that break down our food into molecules that we can re-use to help make new cells and if we water them down we won't get the maximum nutrients from the food we eat. This is such an obvious thing to do I am amazed more people don't do it. So try to avoid diluting them with any drinks whilst you eat and for an hour afterwards.

Chew like a cow (but don't drink the white stuff)

Now I wonder if you have ever counted the number of times you chew each mouthful of food? There is a saying that "you should drink your food". It means chewing each forkful enough times to start breaking down the food. The more you chew the less work your digestive process has to do and the more goodness you will get from what you are eating.

The Dairy Connection

If you remember back to the beginning of my story, I told you about a call I took from an amazing lady who ran a support group. Her name was Judy Geison and she advised me to cut out dairy from my diet immediately and explained briefly why. That simple suggestion changed my life.

I went from being powerless to having a purpose and then my purpose was to confirm or disprove that dairy was very bad for you if you had breast cancer. It became apparent very early on that Judy was right and by the end of that night, I had made the decision to avoid it at all costs.

Very briefly, milk is designed to make a baby calf grow to full size in 9 months. IGF 1, the growth hormone that does this is going to make cells in your body grow quickly too. Not great if you have cancer. I grew up believing that you needed a certain amount of dairy in your diet or your bones would crumble. How wrong was I? The countries in the world that have the highest levels of osteoporosis also have the highest consumption of dairy. The countries that have the lowest levels also consume the lowest amounts. No other species drinks milk after the young have been suckled so why do we? Most of the world is actually intolerant to lactose.

Just chew like a cow, don't copy anything else they do!

Enjoy Your Food

Here is a little experiment for you. Imagine holding a lemon and cutting through it with a sharp knife. Smell that citrusy aroma. Cut a wedge and hold it up to your mouth. Can you taste it before it goes into your mouth? Your saliva is probably flowing by now and this just demonstrates how wonderful the whole process really is. Your saliva is the start of the digestive process and activates your digestive juices to prepare your gut for the food it is about to receive. Ideally, you want to be hungry when you eat and enjoy the smells and sounds of the cooking or preparing process.

If you are eating a meal you don't enjoy then you are really missing out. I think that everything I eat is for a purpose and if I eat too much it won't be good for me. To me, this means that every mouthful I eat has to be a taste delight that nourishes my body. To eat otherwise would be an utter waste.

Acidic Diets

It can get very complicated trying to work out what is and isn't an acidic diet and indeed many books are available on the subject.

In the Western World, we generally eat a high proportion of processed foods and very few people come anywhere near the recommended vegetable and fruit intake. I personally eat anywhere between 12 and 15 a day.

Any processed foods will have an acidic effect on your body and as I have already discussed disease only survives in an acidic body. Logic dictates that by removing these "foods" from our diets and replacing them with whole foods, real foods, ones that come straight from the ground then your body is going to be less acidic

Some foods are acidic but when digested leave an alkaline ash and so are actually good for you. Lemons are a very good example.

Test yourself

You may be interested to know how your body is fairing on the acid/alkaline scale and you can easily find out by purchasing some pH urine or saliva testing strips. Simplex Health makes them. I find testing my urine more reliable and it is very motivating to see how quickly what you eat and drink changes your levels.

The Easy Way

If you are just starting your health journey, or if you haven't already then make things easy for yourself and replace the packaged, processed dead foods with lots of vegetables, ideally with ones that are colourful and try to eat as many as you can with minimal cooking. You will always find someone who says, this or that is good or bad for you, sometimes with scientific backing but stick to these simple suggestions and your health will improve.

KEY ACTION POINTS

- Avoid processed foods like the plague. You have no real idea of the manufacturing processes.
- Eliminate as much sugar from your diet as possible.
- Use the Dirty Dozen and Clean Fifteen Lists.
- If you eat meat check its provenance.
- Add a select few supplements to your daily diet.
- Consider juicing or creating smoothies to replace one meal a day.
- Swap as many unhealthy ingredients in your cupboards for healthier alternatives.
- Chew, chew, chew and keep chewing.
- Enjoy the whole process of shopping, creating, preparing, cooking, serving and eating your meals.
- Avoid dairy.
- Look after your gut.

How To Make These Changes Easy For Yourself

JULIE HARRISON

There is a logic to how I have arranged this book, but do feel free to change around the order of things if you find it suits you better. At the end of the day, this is about your health. So take the information and make it your own.

Your first job

Before you make any changes you really need to sit down and work out what it is you want to achieve. It might be that you just want to lose a couple of pounds, or you might like a complete overhaul. You need to decide.

Take it easy

Why be hard on yourself? Do the small easy changes first. That way you can start to see the positive effects and it will spur you on to achieve greater goals.

Too many people set themselves up for failure by being totally unrealistic about what they can achieve. If for example you have a large meat-eating family and you adore your Sunday joint then trying to be a vegan overnight really isn't going to happen.

Only tell supportive people

Certain people within your family and friends will either think you have lost the plot or be secretly jealous and so go out of their way to stop you from achieving your goals. If you know there are people like that, then the easiest thing is to avoid telling them anything. In a few months' time, they will start to notice the changes in you and no doubt ask and by then you will feel confident and happy with what you have done.

Give yourself a reward

Every day reward yourself, but not with the usual food or drink. Instead, come up with something that is totally decadent to you. It might be as simple as sitting still and watching the sunrise, or a foot rub from a loved one. Whatever it might be, don't forget.

Above all else remember that you are creating a new lifestyle for a new 'you'. This is no fad diet.

The Storm Rumbles On

(more of my story)
Finally, I get to the part of my book
where I explain all that I promised
each time I wrote,
"At the end of this book, I will..."

I do hope I haven't missed anything,
but rest assured that, at the very end,
I will be pointing you to places
where you'll find any answers you need.

Not unexpected

As crazy as it sounds I had always known that I would get cancer. In hindsight, if I had known that, why didn't I change my diet and lifestyle to prevent it? I didn't, because all those years ago I thought I was living a healthy life. Also, I was from the school of thought that thinks medical doctors know best with their surgery, radiotherapy and chemotherapy and the only way of beating the disease was to follow their advice.

Energy Fields and Acupuncture

My quest for true health led me to discover many fabulous therapies and people. For months and years, I experimented and tried many of them.

I have always believed in the body having energy fields and it was recommended that I try acupuncture. Again I fell back to the internet because I didn't know anyone to recommend a good practitioner and I came across Wendy Morrison.

My first appointment with Wendy was amazing. She knows more about me and my medical history than anyone else. She was so professional, thorough and obviously believes that the whole person needs to be looked at rather than individual ailments. This was the first time that I had been treated in this way and my eyes were opened to how everyone should look at their health.

Raw versus cooked foods

The only thing Wendy and I disagreed about was cooked and raw food. From the research I had studied, a diet of mainly raw food—at least 75%, was the way to optimise your health. Cooking, even lightly steaming vegetables kills the enzymes and a lot of the vitamins. Wendy believes in the Chinese way of eating and encouraged me, very strongly to eat more cooked foods.

At this time I was juicing carrots and was turning a little orange, so I agreed to cut down on the raw foods and settled at about 60% raw.

To start with, I went to Wendy once a week and then, twice

a month followed by monthly visits for about a year.

Other Contributory Factors

As you will have discovered by reading my Eight Eye Openers, the healing of the whole person is a lot bigger than I had first thought when I started my journey. I was spending hours each day reading information from books and the internet and my knowledge was expanding at a rate I would love to have happened when I was at school.

At this point, I was starting to bore my friends and family with all these fascinating discoveries I'd made. Like me, before all this, most people I spoke to seemed to think they were doing OK. However, if we're honest, things were usually not right when you look below the surface. How are you doing? Any of this resonating with you? Are you going to make any changes?

Wendy, my acupuncturist, suggested that I had discovered so many things and seemed so passionate about them that I should look at taking things further but when I asked her if she had any ideas she said I needed to think for myself. She wasn't giving me an easy option.

What was wrong BC?

I am often asked what my diet used to be like. I did have a high percentage of fruit and vegetables but nothing was organic. I used a microwave all the time; in the evening I would cook a meal, then clean up and reheat my dinner.

I would cook a weeks' worth of white rice in a plastic bowl in the microwave and keep it in the fridge until needed.

I ate chicken breast and lean minced beef and pork but again not organic. Although I rarely bought any ready meals all grains were refined.

Almost every evening I would have a large glass of wine, sometimes 2. I did drink at least 2 litres of water but this wasn't even pure filtered water, just straight out of the tap.

Next step was to retrain

I made the decision to retrain as a Nutritionist following appointments with an amazing lady called Dilys Gannon-Bone, a colonic therapist. Dilys has had cancer twice, once in her 20's when she was a young doctor and again in her late 30's. The first time she was treated conventionally but the second time she treated herself holistically. She was an inspirational 76, full of life and wisdom. I remember thinking that if I have to work in my 70's I want to be doing something that I love and sharing my knowledge seemed the most logical thing to do.

The search then began for a course that fitted in with everything I had found out. It was at this point that I came across the College of Natural Nutrition and it was like a light bulb had suddenly been lit.

I read a book by *Barbara Wren,* called 'Cellular Awakening' and everything I had learnt over the last eighteen months was all coming together.

Another change in direction

Whilst carrying out other research alongside my nutritionist course, I came to the conclusion that there was more to well being than just nutrition. It was then that I made the decision to become a Natural Health Coach so I could cover these wider areas. I dropped out of the nutritionist course, although many people thought I was mad, but then I had the idea to create a series of health workshops to share my broader knowledge and experience.

Another good reason to trust your instincts and follow your passion in life.

The missing link—Holistic Health

All of my Eye Openers are focusing on the body and mind and how you can change them. I have hinted throughout this book that there is more and indeed when I understood my purpose in life through this process everything clicked into place. Let me tell you a Fairy Tale.

The Fairy Tale—The One

In the very beginning, there was God, or the Universal Energy, or The One, (use whichever sits more comfortably with you).

There was nothing else in the Universe and he/she/it created lots of wonderful things and this went on for Millennia. Things began to get boring and The One decided to split into two and spice things up a little.

The One knew what the other One was thinking and going to do and so things soon became boring again.

The One decided to divide into many, many more Ones, to see if that relieved the boredom.

It didn't.

Then The One had a light bulb moment.

The One decided that they should all forget that they were The One and for them all to be independent of each other.

And that is how most of us think of ourselves.

Some people have remembered that we are all The One. Have you?

My return to The One

The moment I heard this Fairy Tale my world changed. I remembered that we are all one and everything is connected and life became so much easier.

I studied Reiki with Amanda Dobson and became qualified as a Level 2 Reiki Practitioner. Amanda has the most incredible spiritual awareness and has helped me along my journey.

If you ever have the opportunity to try Reiki I strongly urge you to do so. It is a Japanese technique for stress reduction and relaxation that promotes healing through a "laying on of hands", but it is far more than that.

My circle of friends grew and I learnt so much from them. And for that, I am so grateful.

You know who you are...

Health Workshops made easy

The Workshops are now up and running and the feedback

has been truly marvellous. The "side effects" of the changes people are making are profound and wide-ranging. If you need the inspiration to make some of the changes I recommend that you read any of the testimonials on my website.

What next?

Cancer for me has changed my life beyond my wildest dreams in a totally good way, although like all the "bad" experiences in life it doesn't feel like that when you are going through it.

I have been engaged as a motivational/inspirational speaker at numerous events and would love to hear from you if you have a function or event that you would like me to attend.

My 'Deliciously Healthy' recipe book is finished. The idea is to show just how easy it can be to create healthy, tasty and quick meals all the while avoiding dairy, wheat, refined sugar and unfermented soya.

Who knows what is next? But whatever it is it will make me grow as a person and I hold my arms wide open.

I am now no longer frightened of cancer. I feel liberated. I feel safe. I want you to feel the same. I hope my story will inspire you to make changes in your life.

More Help For You

*Tips on where to look
and how you can find
reliable answers
to your questions.*

Recommended Websites to Visit

Be wary of websites funded by pharmaceutical companies. I have found the following to be highly trustworthy:

- **www.mercola.com**—Dr Mercola has the world's most visited natural health website and he has been a physician for two decades, has over a million subscribers and over 300,000 pages of information. A fabulous free resource.
- **www.credence.org**—Phillip Day is an investigative journalist and one of the most knowledgeable and genuine men I have met. His company Credence is an independent research organisation dedicated to reporting contentious issues that may harm the public.
- **www.vitamindcouncil.org**—run by John J Cannell, MD. It is a non-profit organisation educating the public on the importance of vitamin D, sun exposure and health. Some information is free but you can sign up as a paid subscriber to gain more access.
- **www.wddty.com**—What Doctor's Don't Tell You. An online database with more than 23 years of health research and information. They also produce a monthly magazine. The online service is partly free or you can sign up as a paid subscriber to gain full access.
- **www.canceractive.com**—CANCERactive is Britain's Number 1 complementary and integrative cancer charity. There is so much trustworthy information on it.
- **www.getseriouslyhealthy.com**—this is the site I created to help people achieve better health.

There are endless more websites that offer wonderful free information.

A simple test

A good way to assess websites is to find out where the site stands on statins. Conventionally we are told that they reduce cholesterol and protect against heart attacks. Recently levels of acceptable cholesterol have been reduced so that more people became "eligible" to take them.

They are generally harmful and offer very little benefit, and certainly shouldn't be prescribed to as many people as they are, and certainly not as a preventive measure. In one large review by Open Journal of Endocrine and Metabolic Diseases 2013 for every 10,000 people taking the drug, there were

- 307 extra patients with cataracts,
- 23 additional patients with acute kidney failure,
- 74 extra patients with liver dysfunction.

The same study revealed coronary artery and aortic calcification, erectile dysfunction (10 times more common in young men taking the lowest dose), diabetes and even cancer. Are you starting to see why this is a good starting point?

Recommended Reading

- 'Cancer, Why We Are Still Dying for the Truth' by *Phillip Day*
- 'The Essential Guide to Water and Salt' by *F Batmanghelidj MD* and *Phillip Day*
- 'The pH Miracle' by *Robert O Young*
- 'Cellular Awakening' by *Barbara Wren*
- 'The Iodine Crisis' by *Lynne Farrow*
- 'The Biology of Belief' by *Bruce H Lipton*
- 'Living Water' by *Olof Alexandersson*
- 'Hidden Messages In Water' by *Dr Masaru Emoto*
- 'Your Life In Your Hands' by *Jane Plant*
- 'The Rainbow Diet' by *Chris Woollams*
- 'Earthing: The Most Important Health Discovery Ever' by *Clinton Ober*
- 'A Complaint Free World' by *Will Bowen*
- 'Health Wars' by *Phillip Day*
- 'Knockout' by *Suzanne Somers*

JULIE HARRISON

About the Author

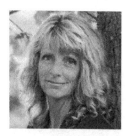

Julie lives in the beautiful South West of England, in Torbay and has done for the whole of her life. She has two grown-up children, a daughter and son, who regularly come home to try out her new recipes and to spend time with their Mum.

Get Seriously Healthy, Julie's company focuses on a varied range of Workshops which she delivers on a weekly basis in Paignton. She has written two other books, 'Deliciously Healthy: quick and easy recipes to improve your health', and 'Deliciously Healthy 2'.

Besides learning about health and wellbeing Julie and her partner, John, love to go for long walks in the countryside and by the sea. Other interests include cycling, sea swimming, Pilates, creating recipes and spending time with her friends and family.

If you could leave a review on Amazon about this book it would be very much appreciated.

Newsletter signup: www.getseriouslyhealthy.com
Facebook: www.facebook.com/nourishmentninja

Improve Your Health

take just one step today...

Take a Workshop with Julie

- Do you want to discover the easiest things you can do to improve your health?
- Are you confused about all the conflicting advice out there?
- Do you want to find out the best and cheapest places to source your supplies?
- Do you want to make divine tasting food, quickly and effortlessly?
- Would you like to find out how to organise your kitchen to save you time & money?
- Fed up with wondering what to cook for dinner?
- Do you know which foods give you the best bang for your buck?
- Would you like some help so that a lot of the hard work is removed?
- Are you curious?
- Are you ready to take control?

Julie's passion is running small Workshops, usually with just 2 or 3 people in her home, so you can see how easy it is to incorporate the various changes into your life. Whether you want a radical overhaul or would prefer to take baby steps, it really doesn't matter. You might be recovering from an illness or just wanting to be as healthy as possible.

Many people do not know who to trust and what to believe, so anything she suggests can easily be researched further and she will point you in the right direction to internet sites you can trust. The important thing is you have started on the road to true health.

When you attend any of her Workshops you will shortcut many years of hard work and learn the tools needed for improving your health. You will learn new, easy and quick recipes, which turn old favourites into health-enhancing delights, all dairy, wheat and refined sugar-free.

The most popular workshop at the moment is her Gut Health Workshop. Learn why it is so important, how you can improve it easily and cheaply and learn how to make some cultured foods and drink. Two hours that could change your life with a FREE goody pack to take home as well. You might even make some new friends.

The Real Health Workshop, which runs most Fridays from 10am until 3pm would be her recommendation to start your journey.

Once you have completed The Real Health Workshop you will probably want to find out more. Due to numerous requests, she created 9 mini workshops which go into more detail on various topics. You don't have to have attended the Real Health Workshop to come along though.

Testimonials

Here's a small selection of testimonials from people who know Julie and have attended her workshops. Much of the information covered in the workshops are shared here in this book.

Phillip Day has this to say about Julie:

"I first met Julie 6 years ago when she attended one of my Workshops. She was uncertain of which route to take so that her body could heal from one of life's most serious illnesses - natural or conventional. Thankfully she decided to change her diet and lifestyle. Over the following years, she has kept in contact with me and I have been extremely impressed with her wealth of knowledge and the way she has turned her life around. The Thermogram images she has done yearly certainly back this up. Julie's passion now is helping others and she has created 10 Health Workshops to educate and assist others to take control too. I can highly recommend them if you want some practical guidance along your own journey."

Wendy Mason from Torquay:

"Julie's Real Health Workshop was a profound, nourishing and stimulating day for me and she shines as a beautiful healthy example of the results of living altruistically in body, mind and spirit. She is so committed and dedicated to sharing something wonderful and magical that she has discovered borne out of her own manifesting of cancer. She is generous in the extreme, working as hard as she does to share her discoveries and knowledge."

Jane MacNamara from Abbotskerswell:

·"Julie at Improve Your Health is an amazing and very knowledgeable and inspiring lady. The workshops are brilliant and very informative and relaxed and I would highly recommend. Enjoyed the very tasty lunch of Raw Pad Thai salad and Raw Key Lime Pie (we did it with lemons and it was delicious). Feeling happier and healthier."

Hazel Self from Torquay:

"I have attended one of Julie's Real Health Workshops and it was an absolutely fantastic day. I couldn't believe the amount of information we were given! Julie's enthusiasm is infectious and her level of knowledge is incredible. Julie is clearly passionate about her subject and it is clear that she wants to share this knowledge and passion to improve the health and well-being of others. One of the aspects I particularly liked was the fact that Julie kept the energy of the workshop flowing with different activities and sessions. I didn't want the day to end! The value for money was exceptional; this is a workshop jam-packed and busting at the seams with content. Although there is a lot of learning, Julie's delivery is natural and she makes everything easy to understand. Julie feels like a friend from the start and it is easy to warm to her relaxed yet confident style. I left the workshop feeling energised, informed and excited. The workshops are ideal for all levels of knowledge and those new to taking steps to improve their health shouldn't hesitate—everyone was made to feel welcome and everyone learnt a lot. I would highly recommend Julie and her Real Health Workshop to "anyone! A great day is in store!"

Jacqueline Horsfall from Torquay:

"I really cannot recommend Julie's Gut Health Workshop highly enough! The morning workshop surpassed all expectations. I came away armed with knowledge, inspiration and practical skills and tips to start my new journey in discovering how I can achieve greater health, energy and vitality to support myself during the next chapter of my life. I really didn't have any idea just how important gut health is! Thankfully I do now! Julie has extensive knowledge and shares it in a clear, concise, easy to follow manner. Her passion on the subject shines through. I felt inspired and motivated. Julie kindled an excitement in me, which sadly has been very lacking in recent years, to open myself to learning more about the choices available to us with foods, and to experimenting with alternative food choices to gain greater gut health, and overall health and happiness benefits. I am definitely booking in next for her "Raw Food Lessons" Workshop."

Chris Avery from Torquay:

"I'm in much better shape than I was when I came to your workshop.

My cough is almost gone and my eyesight has improved greatly. So much so that now I'm wearing glasses that were prescribed for me 7 or 8 years ago. The macular degeneration that was developing in my right eye has now totally gone."

Dan Nuttall from Paignton:

"Helen and I both took a lot of great advice away from your workshop and have implemented real change into our lives.

You'll be pleased to hear we have a regular batch of Kombucha on rotation. All the scoby's can be traced back to the one you gave us! We really enjoy the taste and the pro-biotic benefit of the drink. I'm going to have to buy some more mason jars as it quickly runs low, despite being on a permanent brewing cycle.

We have bought a Jason Vale "Fusion" juicer and regularly juice / make smoothies. I'm a huge advocate of both juicing and smoothies and have got my mother into it after we invited her round for juices and smoothies of varying concoction!

Sugar—in its refined form—is completely out of the household. The only source is a bag for brewing the Kombucha. I now take zero sugar in tea, coffee and never add it to cereal or anything else. It's a pleasant surprise just how fine everything tastes without sweetening it; it goes to show how much we have been conditioned in our society. The only source of sugar is the naturally occurring fructose in the fruit we eat. There are no biscuits, crisps, chocolate, puddings, cakes in the house and the only time we indulge is if we're guests at someone's house or similar.

I still train hard on the bike and have noticed an increase in speed and endurance. I put this is partly down to the changes I have made thanks to your guidance. The only downside is an ever-changing wardrobe, as I keep shaving off the pounds! I was a size larger about four to five years ago and now I'm almost on the edge of extra small! (That's great for cyclists though!)"

Rebecca Box from Torquay:

"Thank you, Julie, you have helped make this time of transition much easier for me by sharing your knowledge and enthusiasm in such a loving and professional way.

Attending your workshop has been amazing for me. I am loving making and drinking the Kombucha. My brownies have improved and I've even made cashew nut ice-cream to go with them. Fermented vegetables are improving too."

Printed in Great Britain
by Amazon

23081870R00073